Aloe Vera Manual

Author

Mervyn George Bryan Dip. VTCT

(Health and Nutrition - Holistic Therapies & Swedish Massage VTCT)
(Aloe Naturopath) (Member IASC)
Researcher Nutritional Medicine
Director - Health Life Centre
Director Health Life Publications

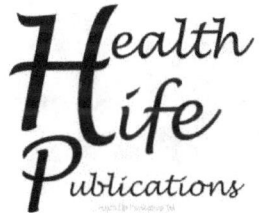

http://www.healthlifepublications.com

Advisor and Aloe distributor:-

Warwick Bryan RMN SEN
Complimentary Therapist
(Nutritionalist, Naturopathic, Cpdc)

Contents

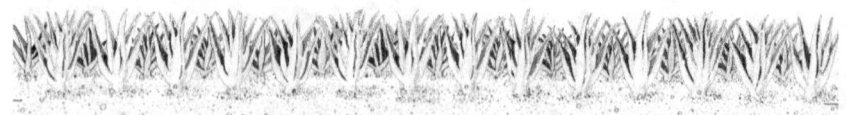

The Author and Contributors

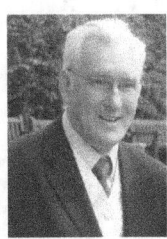

- Mervyn George Bryan, the author became interested in health issues because of his personal ill health

- He has had stress and allergy related asthma since a young child

Mervyn Bryan

- In 1979 he developed a duodenal ulcer and was given the wrong dosage of a drug with the resultant agonising side effects

- In 1983 he was introduced to holistic nutritional medicine

- Aloe Vera helps his body to correct the imbalances that were causing his duodenal ulcer

- Since then he has been promoting proactive nutritional health

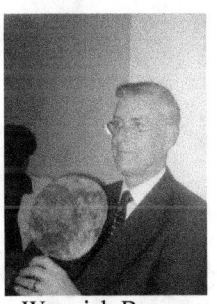

- Mervyn introduced his findings to his brother Warwick, a qualified nurse

- His brother calls Aloe Vera a "Red Indian Witch Doctors Brew"

Warwick Bryan

- But out of frustration and amid great pain tries it. WOW!
- Warwick becomes an instant convert

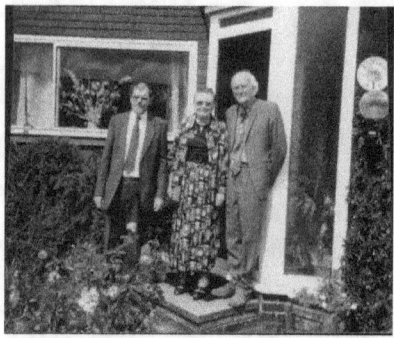

John, Margaret and husband Ken

- Margaret Rosier our aunt was a qualified nurse and trainer and joined them in their research

- She was a retired nursing teacher and had been head of Staffordshire's St John's ambulance service

- Margaret's son John a qualified English teacher has helped edit the work

The Author and this book.

This book is the result of my life work since March of 1983, when my family and I were first introduced to the use of Aloe Vera for its healing benefits.

It became amply clear that little was at that time understood about this miracle of nature. Since then my brother and I have done all we could to remedy this situation.

First I began to research at the Birmingham City Public Library, writing to all the Aloe companies, organisations and individuals I could find, and eventually became a member of the *"International Aloe Science council"*.

Today my brother and I continue to lecture, and teach all who request our services.

Our involvement in the Aloe Vera industry includes introducing the product to a number of companies which today thrive in the British Aloe industry.

However, we are concerned at the lack knowledge and amount of misinformation which has accumulated concerning Aloe Vera. In the following pages you will find a simple to understand text information showing why Aloe Vera is needed, what Aloe Vera is, how it works and how it should be used. All this information is backed up by a source list at the end of the book and index.

More information about the way Aloe Vera works at cellular level to aid our body is becoming available each day. The latest information included in this book will convey to you in an easy to understand way, the basic information that science now possesses, proving that Aloe Vera does work.

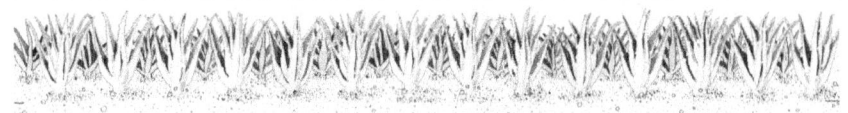

I am grateful to my brother Warwick a qualified nurse, and to John, for their help with this book.
The following pages have progressed through various stages of evolution to become what we hope is the most thorough background on this subject.

Author. *Mervyn Bryan.*

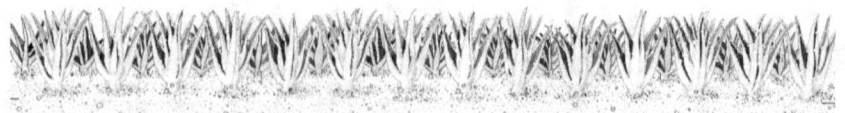

How it started

I had a number of health problems which I had inherited from birth and added to during my life.

- Allergies
- Asthma
- Eczema
- Stress related skin problems
- Duodenal Ulcer

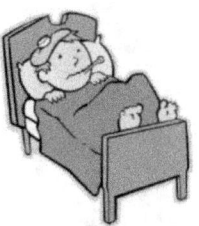

Our church minister knew of my problems and suggested I use Aloe Vera.

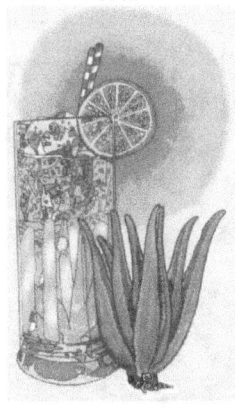

I took his advice and have not looked back since.

- Within hours of drinking the recommended dose, the pain from my ulcer lessened.

- Using it on my skin my eczema disappeared

- My health simply improved in every way

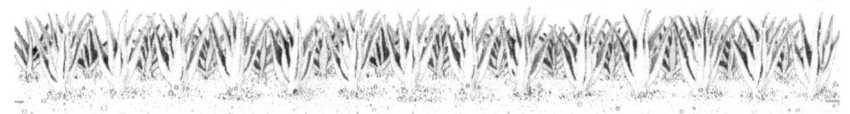

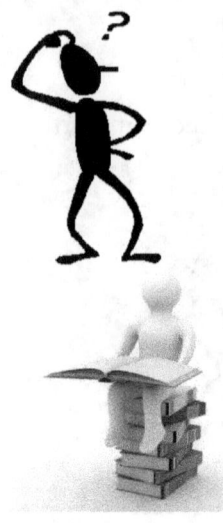

I couldn't understand why the National Health Service wasn't using this wonderful product.

I was soon to find out!

Realising the potential of this herbal vegetable in 1983 I started to do research in the Birmingham city library and at the university regarding this phenomena. A process that occupies my time to this very day.

Because Aloe Vera is a natural herbal vegetable, just like the onion or garlic, its cousins. It cannot be patented. Hence the pharmaceutical firms could make little money out of it.

Over the years we have accumulated files of information from both scientific and lay testimonial sources. Also from government sources, laboratory testing, hospital, clinical and personal use, which have all added to our appreciation. We found that there are many scientifically controlled tests which show the efficacy of the Gel obtained from this *"Miracle of Nature"*.

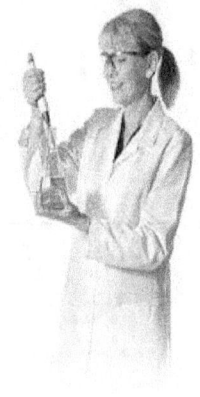

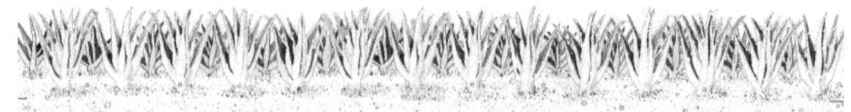

During this period of time our family, friends, and colleagues have tried and practically tested every major Aloe Vera Gel and Juice available in the UK, U. S. A., Australia and New Zealand.

The results have varied greatly, according to the apparent purity of the product. It is the scientific results of these experiences, and our enthusiasm for Aloe Vera which we will share in the following pages.

What is Aloe Vera?

The Aloe Vera plant
A brief description

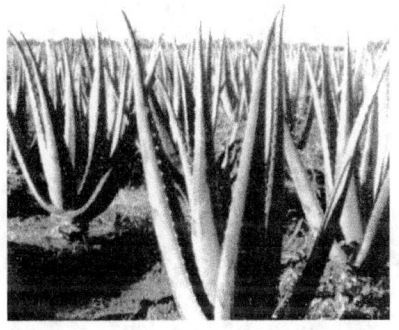

"Let food be your medicine and medicine be your food".
Hippocrates.

Of all the nearly two million documented species in the botanical kingdom, Aloe Vera (Aloe Barbadensis) is probably one of the best known for its historic therapeutic use. Today more and more research is being directed toward this one herbal, Aloe Vera gel.

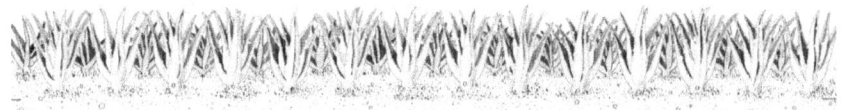

Wherever it is available for use, it becomes a household name as part of the family medicine cabinet and daily diet.

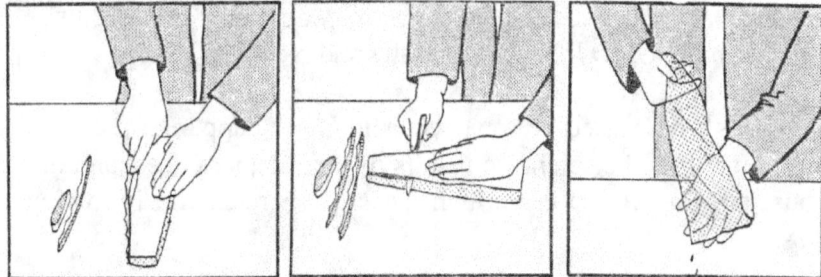

The Aloe leaf structure is made up of three parts:-

1. **Rind** - *the outer protective layer.*
2. **Sap** - *a layer of bitter fluid which helps protect the plant from animals*
3. **Mucilage Gel** - *the inner part of the leaf that is filleted out to make Aloe Vera Gel.*

Aloe Vera (inner gel) contains Amino Acids and nutrients that the human body needs for healing purposes. Many of which the body cannot manufacture for itself.

For the gel from the centre of the leaf of this plant to attain maturity, it requires at least four years growth stimulated by a warm moist breeze. When filleted it forms a near clear fillet which can be held in the hand. Each leaf has to be tested for maturity and harvested separately by hand and filleted within hours of harvesting. The cold stabilisation of the gel has only been made available to us because of modern hygienic methods and an understanding of the plant's chemistry.

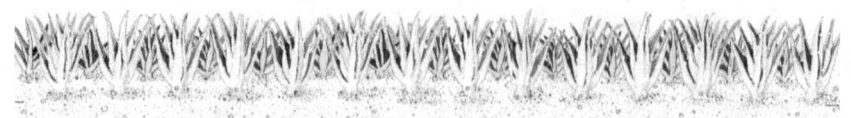

The name of the plant helps describe to us what it tastes like.
The word Aloe stems from the Arabic source-word "aloe-h",
meaning "shining bitter substance, and is pronounced "AI-law-oe"
The name Vera is Latin in origin and gives the meaning of truth. It
is pronounced "Vee-rah". Hence a literal translation of the name
ALOE VERA would be, **"The true bitter plant'** :

Although Aloe Vera's origins can be traced to areas of the Eastern
Mediterranean, it also grows all over the world in the tropical belt.
Parts of China, Malaya, Burma, India, Australia, Arabia, Israel,
Egypt, Spain, Portugal, the West Indies. as well as central and
north America, where it can be found in Costa Rica, Guatemala,
Mexico, and in the states of Texas, Florida and California.

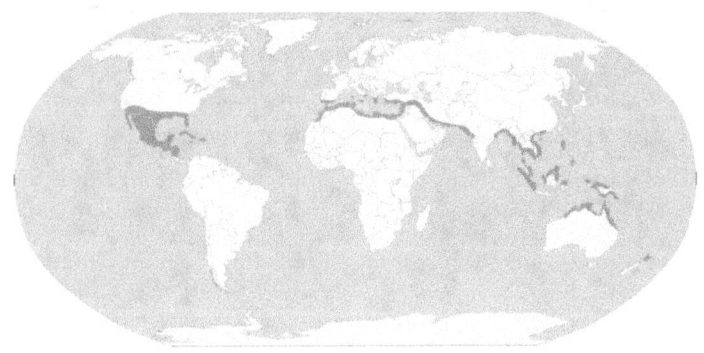

The dark areas of the world map above show the areas that
Aloe can grow in

Aloe Vera is the botanical named ALOE BARBADENSIS
MILLER.

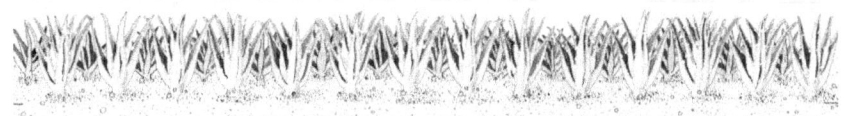

1. The Gel of which we are speaking has the American Chemical Society Number 8001-97-S. It is registered as a vegetable food.

2. The yellow sap {Aloin) also known as Bitter Aloes has the number 85507- 69-3

The yellow sap should not be mixed up with the Gel, as they have a totally different chemical makeup and action.

The gel obtained from a mature leaf of Aloe Vera is a:-

CONCENTRATE LIVING
POTENTISED BOTANICAL LIQUID,
with MULTI VITAMIN, MINERAL, AMINO ACID,
and ENZYME Gel with NATURAL SUGARS IN IT
whose synergistic balance and Biological
activity is activated by
LIVING ELECTROLYTES

The Aloe leaf contains over **75** nutritional components and **200** other compounds, including **20** minerals, **18** amino acids and **12** vitamins.

It is an all-round Nutritional Storehouse.

- **Vitamins** - essential for good health - including C,E,Beta Carotene, B12

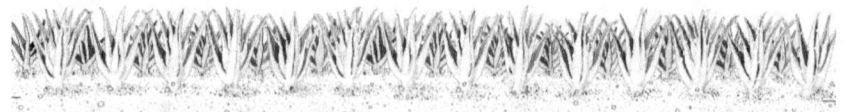

- **Minerals** - the building blocks of the body - including magnesium, manganese, zinc, copper, chromium, calcium, sodium, potassium, iron.

- **Amino Acids** - 20 out of the 22 required by the body as the building blocks for protein and 7 out of the 8 that the body cannot manufacture itself

- **Sugars** - including long chain polysaccharides that help boost the immune system

- **Enzymes** - the chemical switches that activate cell activity -and help break down and digest food

- **Plant Sterols** - that act as powerful anti-inflammatory agents

- **Lignin** - a woody substance that helps Aloe penetrate the skin

- **Saponins** - soapy substances with an anti-microbial effect

- **Anthraquinone**s - powerful natural painkillers

- **Salycylic Acid** - anti-inflammatory, helps break down dead tissue

To obtain an effective Aloe Vera Gel that is beneficial to the body it is harvested in the following order.

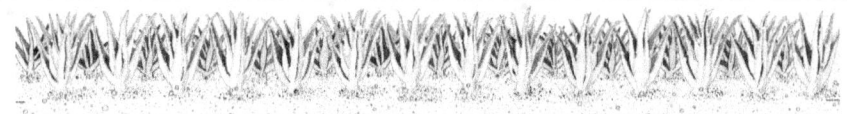

- After at least 4 years of growth the outer leaves are harvested

- The harvested leaves must go to the processing plant immediately to reduce oxidization

- The inner gel is separated from the rind and the sap washed off

- In the tubs the natural antioxidants are added and mixed into the gel

- It is then packaged ready for transit to sale sites

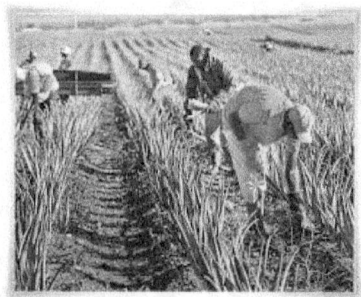
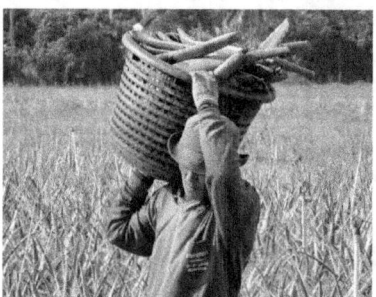
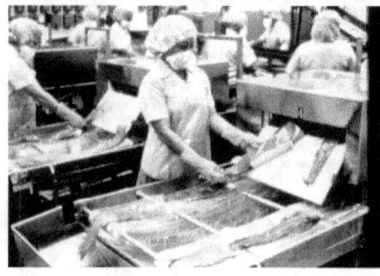
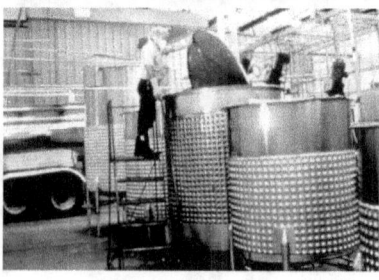

The many names of Aloe Vera help us understand its uses

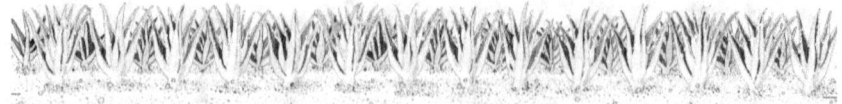

Aloe Vera has been called by many names, which relate to the use it has been put too in various countries. Some of these are:-

- *No Need of Doctor,*
- *Miracle plant,*
- *Band Aid plant,*
- *Medicine plant,*
- *Healing plant,*
- *Magic medicine plant,*
- *Nature's panacea,*
- *First-aid house plant,*
- *The Super plant,*
- *Fountain of Youth plant,*
- *Nature's own medicine plant,*
- *Ancient key to health and beauty,*
- *Burn plant,*
- *Wound healing plant,*
- *The Health giving plant,*
- *Trinity or Bible plant,*
- *Heaven's blessing plant,*
- *Plant of Life,*
- *Mystical plant,*
- *Nature's blessing plant,*
- *Bitter Aloes plant,*
- *Man's natural medical chest,*
- *First Aid plant,*
- *Immortality plant,*

- *Wand of Heaven, and*
- *Flow of Life.*

In Spain it is called ...Seville
Malaysia ...Jadam
China ...Lui-hui
Portugal ...Erva Babosa
Jamaica ...Sinkle Bible (It's in the Bible)
West Indies ...Aloes
Egypt ...Wand of Heaven
Hawaii ...Miracle plant
Japan ...No need of doctor
Sanskrit ...Ghrita-Kumars
India ...Ghee-Guar Ka-Palhtha

The History of Aloe Vera

3500 years of documentation of its medical uses
Pictures on Egyptian archaeological sites
1750 BC Sumarian clay tablets
1500 BC Paperus Ebers describes its medical uses

Its documented ancient uses include:-

- On wounds
- Digestive problems
- Burns
- Skin care
- Haemorrhoids

Historical Users include:-

- Romans,
- Greeks,
- Algerians
- Indians,
- Chinese,

- Jews,
- Moroccans,
- Tunisians,
- Arabians,

Among its best known users were:-

- Solomon,
- Alexander the Great,
- Cleopatra,
- Disciples of Jesus Christ,

- Roman legions,
- Marco Polo,
- Columbus
- British Army in India.

In the case of Cleopatra, it is said to have attributed to her beauty. This is because of her practice of bathing in a mixture of goat's milk and the Aloe Gel.

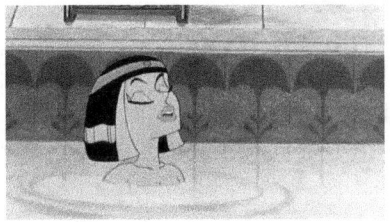

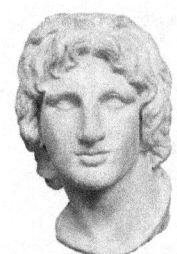

Alexander the Great used it to great effect in the treating of the wounds of his soldiers. Records indicate that this stopped infection, eased pain and speeded up the healing process.

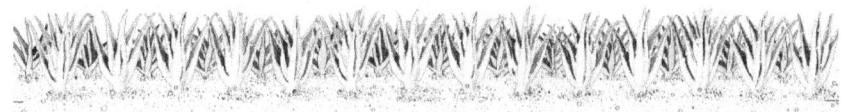

It is mentioned in 5 places in the **Bible** Numbers 24:6, Psalms 45:8, Proverbs 7:17, Song of Solomon 4:14, and in John 19:39 where it speaks of Aloe being used on Christ's body after His death.

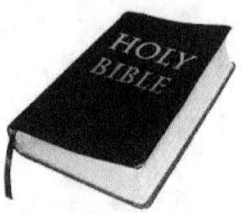

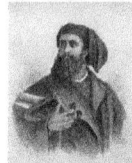

Marco Polo noted its use in China, stating that it had long been an established ingredient of Chinese medicine. The Chinese spoke of its life giving forces.

The Spanish found the native Americans using it. They called it the Plant of Immortality.

In Japan Aloe is *called "No need of doctor*

In India Sir George Watt, a physician in the British Army in the early twentieth century, credited Aloe Vera, (Ghee-guar ka-palhtha) with no less than 43 different medicinal uses. Even as late as the Burma campaign, 1944, British soldiers were trained in its use.

In Africa it is used as a body deodorant, when hunting wild animals. Some tribes use it as a cleanser at times of sickness.

It was during the treatment of radiation burns from X-rays, in the 1930's, that Aloe Vera was resurrected by modern medical science. Burns from early ex-ray machines seemed almost incurable, until doctors tried the fresh gel of Aloe Vera on their patients. More recent research has shown Aloe to be the best treatment for radiation burns.

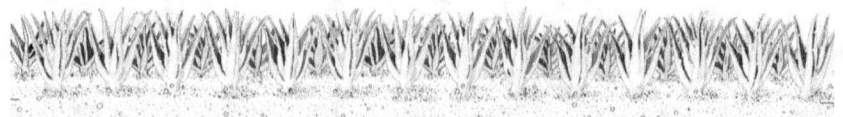

Aloe Vera and your Doctors Prescriptions

It is often thought that we cannot use Aloe Vera alongside doctors drugs. However, this is a complete miss understanding. In most cases the use of the vegetable herb Aloe Vera can enhance the ability of the drug in its work.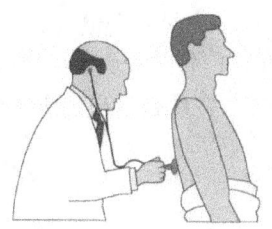

Even when you do not feel that benefit, digestion and immune responses will benefit. So using Aloe as a supplement to your normal diet will always be a benefit. After all, Aloe Vera is a vegetable.

Because Aloe Vera has healing benefits, diabetics often find that once taking it, they are able to reduce their intake of insulin because of the benefits to the pancreas.

Because Aloe Vera helps promote oxygen uptake and normal cell activity, some cancer sufferers find it helps lessen radiation burns.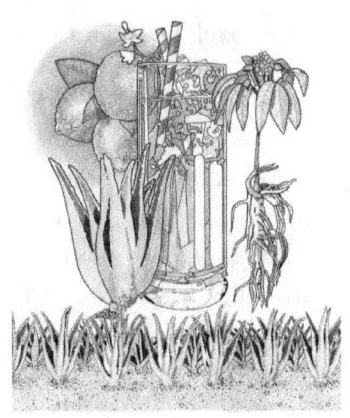

One of the greatest benefits that Aloe Vera users report is that when they take Aloe Vera on a regular basis, the side effects of their doctors prescription lessen and in many cases disappear.

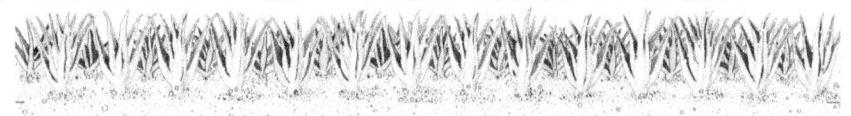

Aloe Vera as your Active Medicine

Many people find that using Aloe Vera benefits their overall health. It is scientifically understood to activate and normalize cell activity throughout the body. Dr. Plackett's research verified this activity of Aloe Vera as being the main reason that Aloe Vera has the reputation in the medical fields.

Dr Plaskett is a research biologist and developed among other things, instant tea and coffee. When we first met him, he was running a mail order supplement company. However he was suffering from a duodenal ulcer. So, naturally we introduced Him to Aloe Vera. He started to use it and found it of benefit.

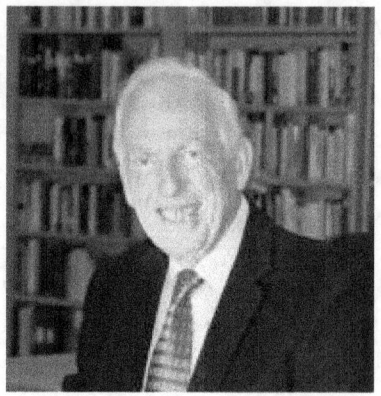

This was back in the mid 1980's when we were the only importers of Aloe Vera into this country. He added Aloe Vera to his mail order list.

His reputation in the industry is such that he was given a large sum by the Trebor foundation to investigate Aloe Vera. Most of the scientific statements in this publication are from the resultant scientific papers that he produced.

Today he runs the Plaskett International College. UK.

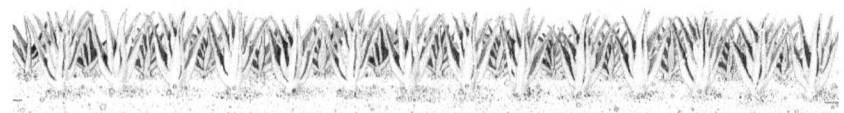

We mention this to enable you to realise that the many of the claims made for Aloe Vera are not just here say or person testimony, but do in fact have scientific support. In fact it has been said that more scientific research has been conducted on this herbal vegetable which has helped establish its reputation.

Aloe Vera and the human cell

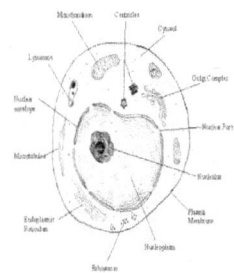

1. All living things are composed of one or more cells.

2. Cells are the fundamental units of structure and function in a living organism.

3. Cells arise only from pre-existing cells by a process of division.

Scientific study by the French investigator Francois-Vincent Raspail in 1825 and later by the German physiologist Virchow in 1855 demonstrates that all existing cells came from already existing cells by the process of division. Later the famous scientist Louis Pasteur with his bacteria experiments further demonstrated that:-

- Existing cells could only come from pre-existing cells.
- The cell within its protective membrane is a chemical factory of complex synergism.
- The loss of any one component would destroy its ability to function.
- When a cell stops functioning as it is designed to do for any reason, ill health prevails.

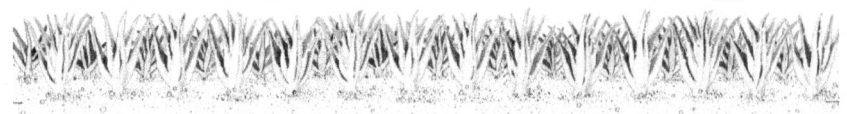

- The naturopathic principles supported in this publication are based on the scientific facts as seen in the biochemical reactions known as metabolism.

- Through this process each cell seeks to maintain a dynamic equilibrium which supports a balance in health.

- If anything interferes with its vital functions and the ability of the cell to function correctly is destroyed, it then affects the adjoining cells and if nothing is done to correct the balance, ill health and then eventually death prevails.

The Cell - Life force Triangle

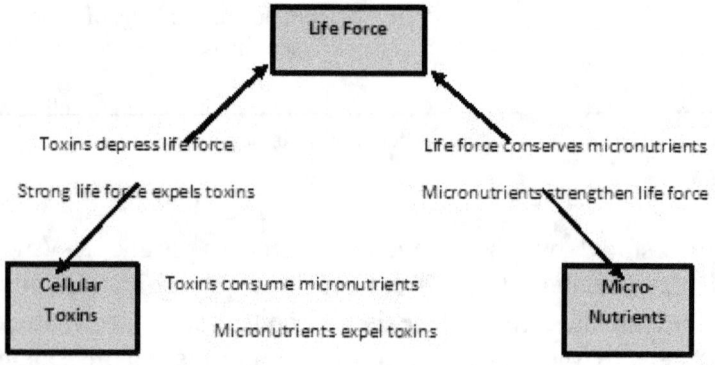

- Nutrients enter the cell by way of osmotic action through the cell membrane

- Nutrients put to work in the cell to provide the necessary chemical activities vital for health

- Chemical processes produce toxins

- Toxins expelled from cell

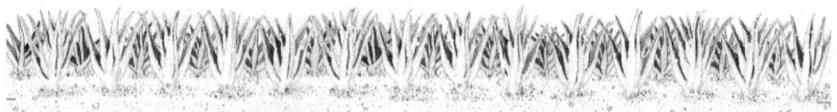

Because of the chemical makeup of Aloe Vera, it helps to reduce surface tension and support the osmotic action that encourages uptake of nutrients and the expelling of toxins. In short Aloe Vera helps the human cells to work correctly.

Assimilation and Elimination

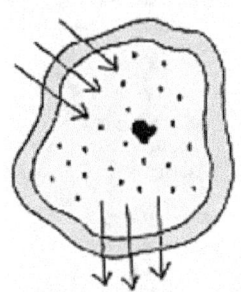 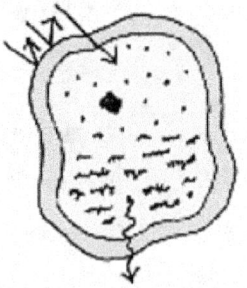

Healthy Cell

Nutrients can be easily assimilated and elminated

Unhealthy Cell

Assimilation and elimination are vastly inhibited

Healthy cells = healthy body.

Cells

Tissues

300 Billion
New Cells
Organs   Every Day

200 Million
Systems   Per Minute

Body

The body not only needs to maintain the health of existing cells, but also it needs to provide the nutrients necessary for reproduction of cells.

Aloe Vera helps in both these processes. Hence it helps the body to correct existing problems and ward off new ones.

How and Why Aloe Vera Gel works

Action of Aloe	Aloe components responsible	Reported medical conditions benefited
Anti -Inflammatory	Solicylates Bradykininase Anti-histamine Plant Sterols - Sitosterol - Luteol	Arthritis, Burns, Dental Surgery, Diabetes, Inflammatory Digestive disorders (Peptic Ulcers), Hepatitis, Otolaryngology, Pain (indirectly) Radiation Burns, Skin disease, Sports Injuries & Wounds
Healing (Mitogenic) [Cell regeneration by division]	Glucomannan Plant Hormones (Auxins & Gibberellins)	Arthritis, Burns, Dental Surgery, Digestive Disorders, Otolaryngology, Radiation Burns, Skin disease, Sports Injuries & Wounds
Immune stimulant	Glucomannan With Immune Cell number increase by the mitogenic effect	Resistance to Infections, Bacterial, Fungal, Viral; Arthritis, Dentistry, Diabetes, Hepatitis, Tumours, Wounds
Digestive A cell stimulant effect increasing secretion of digestive juices	Glucomannan and Aloin With Cell number increase by the mitogenic effect, expulsion of toxins allowing absorption of nutrients	Digestive disorders including Peptic Ulcers
Anaesthetic	Anti- inflammatory and Cell regeneration	Actual direct relief of pain
Antiseptic (Exudate only [Aloin])	Anthraquinones Anthrones Chromones	Direct killing of Bacteria & Fungi

Aloe Vera and Skin Care

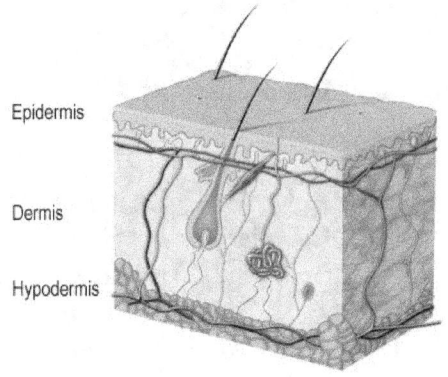

Aloe Vera works by osmosis to penetrate all layers of the skin, enabling its nutritional healing and eliminating activities to do their work.

Today Aloe Vera is recognised for its beauty therapy.

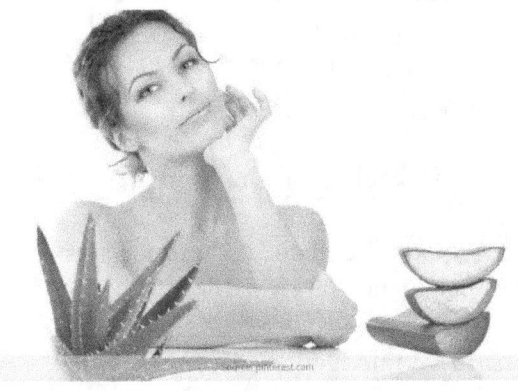

Today hundreds of companies include Aloe Vera in their skin and beauty products. However, much of this is sales hype, as most of them include so little Aloe that it has very little if any effect.

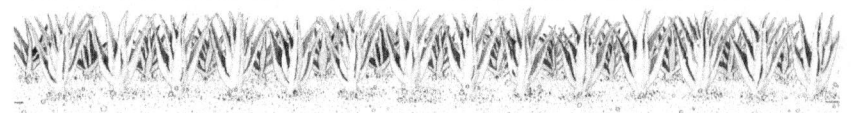

To be certain of the efficacy of the product, Aloe Vera should be the largest constituent part of the product.

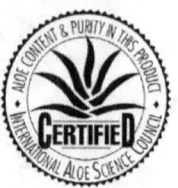

Look for the seal of approval from the **Aloe Science Council** on the product.

- The Aloe Vera Science Council test the magnesium and calcium content as well as the Bonded Amine Column (HPLC Ratio} which shows the efficacy of any product.

- If this seal of approval is on the product you can be certain of its quality.

- The above components were chosen because they occur naturally in Aloe Vera Gel, and are relatively stable and predictable, being difficult to falsify and vary little from location to location or time of year. Finally, they can be assayed easily by most laboratories.

Polysaccharide Components

As with all living plant life there are complex molecular chain substances which makes the plant what it is.

These polysaccharide compounds are very complex. There are 3 basic types of polysaccharides found naturally in the inner Aloe Vera gel of the Aloe Vera leaf.

1. *B 1-4 glucomannan*: This group of polysaccharides is most closely related to cellulose. It is from this group that the polysaccharide known as Acemannon was isolated. This

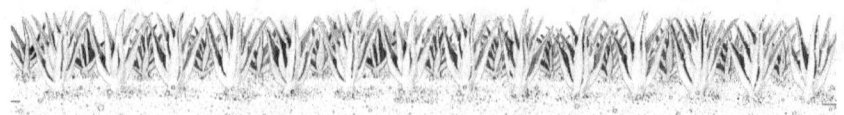

group is believed to be largely responsible for many of the Aloe leaf's special properties.

2. *Galactose base polysaccharides*: This group is similar to most natural gums such as carrageenan gum (*Irish moss*) which belong to this group of polysaccharides.

3. *Acid polysaccharides*: These are polysaccharides with an acid group attached. *Pectin* is a well-known chemical of this group.

The following table demonstrates the solids contents that could be expected from the variously accepted forms of Aloe Vera Juice production.

Method Of Preparation	pH	Aloin (ppm)	(%) H_2O	(%) Solids	Total
Hand-filleting	4.27	6	99.25	0.48	
Roller	4.30	32	99.61	0.39	
Leaf Splitter	4.24	18	99.61	0.42	
Whole Leaf	4.09	1	98.62	1.38	

Any product with an aloin factor of greater than 6% is not suitable for internal consumption, hence the two methods usually utilised for the preparation of Aloe Vera Juice is hand-filleting and whole leaf production.

The best Aloe Vera to use

Hand filleting is the most expensive method but results in the product containing the best balance of nutrients and active components of any method.

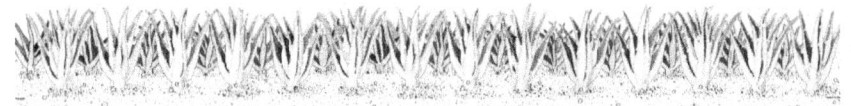

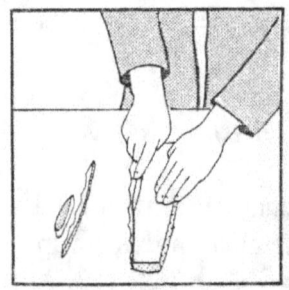 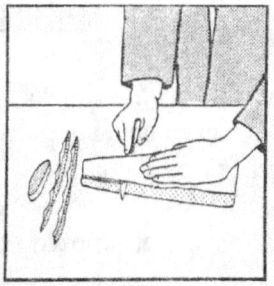 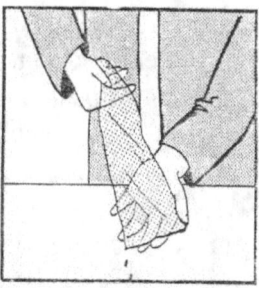

The leaves are opened by hand and the gel and the rind / skin is separated from the inner gel. The inner gel is washed to remove the aloin (yellow sap) and the gel is then liquidised and placed in sterile containers ready to bottle.

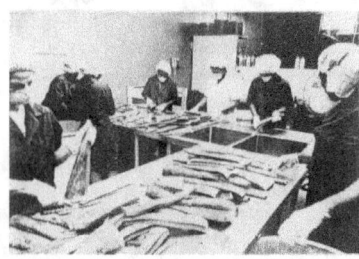 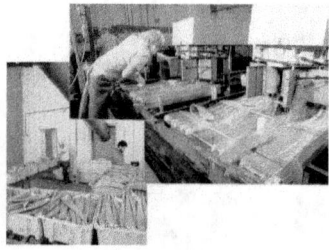

The whole leaf method utilises pressing the leaves between rollers under pressure which produced a juice which then has to be filtered to remove the aloin. As you have seen from the chart, rolling the leaves produces a product with an aloin count of 32 which has to be reduced by active filtering. This filtering process not only reduces the aloin count, but absorbs some other ingredients, which diminishes the natural nutrient and activity of the end product.

Hence we would suggest that for internal use we obtain the hand filleted variety.

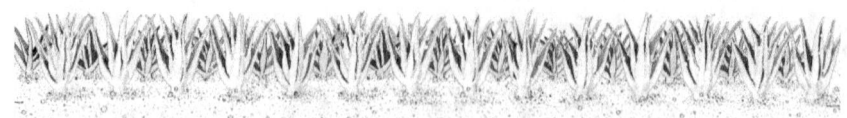

Freeze Dried Aloe Vera

Tablets and Capsules or Aloe Vera in powdered form

People have become accustomed to taking tablets. As many people don't like the bitter taste of Aloe Vera, some companies have freeze dried Aloe Vera into a powder. This process produces an easily transported product that can be added into products. This is usually the source of Aloe Vera used in the many products available in the general stores.

- From a business point of view this may appear a good way of obtaining Aloe Vera to use.

- Freeze drying reduces the valuable nutrient ingredients and activities of the end product.

- It removes the liquid which is an active component in the Aloe Vera. The liquid form of Aloe Vera is important as it clears the digestive tract of unwanted toxins which results in a greater uptake of nutrients.

Recently in the UK there has been a product on the market that is nicely flavoured and contains Aloe Vera Gel and a Freeze Dried version to boost the Aloe Vera strength in the product. This product is bottled in normal plastic containers which results in enzymic activity taking place, thus reducing the positive effects of the product available from 100% varieties. To stabilise Aloe Vera to provide the greatest possible value to the body, it needs to be stored in chemical resistant containers.

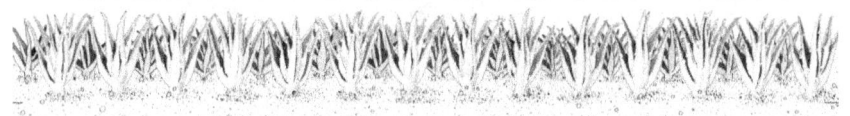

Where to get Aloe Vera from.

It is not the purpose of this manual to promote any one companies product. However from the information given above, it is clear that not all Aloe Vera products will be the same.

Below are some pointers which will help the reader to find the best active Aloe Vera available to use.

a) Does it say it is 100% stabilised Aloe Vera on the label

b) Is it in a chemically and light resistant container? Usually a white plastic or a dark glass bottle, or a specially made plastic container.

c) Does it have on the label the Aloe Science Council seal of approval?

d) In the UK products that meet these descriptions can be found in Health Food stores, by mail order and by direct sales.

e) The most potent products that we have found is one that is sold by direct sales trained Multi Level marketing agents from an international firm. Their product meets all the standards mentioned and have the largest range of high potency Aloe Vera products available.

f) Finally, you can tell the real product by its natural slightly bitter taste and you get what you pay for.

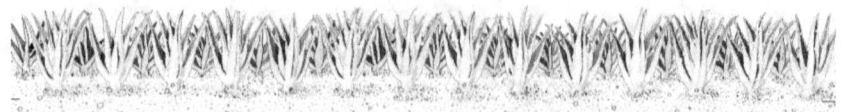

Reported Medical Conditions

Below is a list of medical conditions that doctors and users alike say that Aloe Vera has helped them or their patients with. We make no claims that you will personally find Aloe Vera to be a miracle cure. But having read this publication, I am sure you will realise that Aloe Vera has both scientific and testimonial support for its use.

Usually it is best to use the product at the recommended quantity for at least three months to obtain the best results.

You've got nothing to lose, try it for yourself and see what happens. 99% of users are satisfied.

Aching Muscles	Acid Reflux Disease
Acne	Arthritis
Asthma	Boils
Burns	Cancer
Cholesterol	Chronic Fatigue Syndrome (CFS)
Constipation	Crohns Disease
Cuts and Wounds	Dermatitis
Diabetes	Diverticulum
Dry Skin	Eczema
Fibromyalgia	Genital Herpes
Gout	Gums
Hair Loss	Hay fever
Hemorrhoids and	HIV
Bleeding Piles	
Hypertension	Interstitial Cystitis
Irritable Bowel	Joint Pain
Syndrome (IBS)	

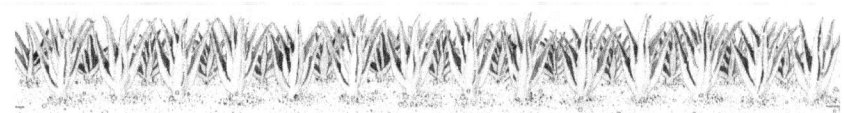

Kidney Stones	Liver Spots
Lupus	Malaria
Migraine	Milia
Nappy Rash	Pancreatitis
Psoriasis	Rheumatism
Scalds	Scars
Sinus Problems	Skin Reactions from Radiotherapy
Skin Spots	Spastic Colon
Stretch Marks	Sunburn
Tendinitis	Trigeminal Neuralgia
Ulcerative Colitis	Ulcers of the Mouth
Ulcers of the Skin	Ulcers of the Stomach
Varicose Veins	

Aloe Vera and Naturopathy

First of all let us define Naturopathy. This is the utilisation of natural means, means provided by nature, to aid in being healthy, obtaining or regaining a balance in health.

This can be by way of the use of:-

➢ Herbs

➢ Vitamin and Mineral Supplements

➢ Massage - medical manipulation

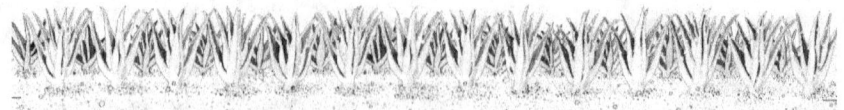

A definition of naturopathy, otherwise known as healing by nutrition would invoke the saying

"We are what we eat."

Nutritionist's agree that the diet we use in western society, by and large, does not, nor can it possibly meet the total nutritional needs of our body. The reasons for this include the fact that all foods in Western society are to some degree affected by modern agricultural and distribution practices.

These lessen the mineral content of vegetables and grains which we eat and feed to the animals.

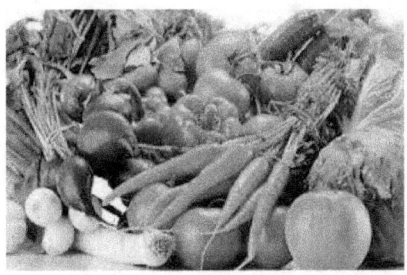

The time it takes for vegetables and grains to travel from harvest to resale can vary from a few days to years, dependent on the item and the market place at the time. As all vegetables begin to lose nutritional value within hours of being harvested, much of that we consume is lessened in its nutritional value beyond that deficiency modern farming techniques have already caused.

There are two ways in which we can help overcome these deficiencies in our food production.

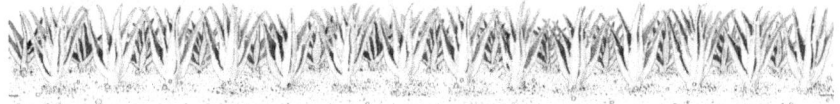

Eat organic foods and obtain food direct from the grower within hours of harvesting.

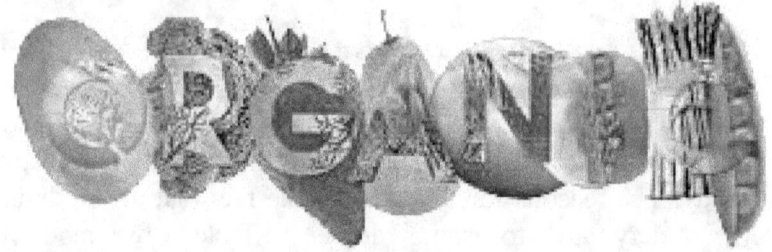

As neither of these, in many instances is practical, a compromise can be the use of frozen vegetables and fruits or naturally dried fruits etc. with a guarantee of freezing or drying within six hours of harvesting.

Another problem with the diet we have is that of white bread and pastries which tend to glue up the digestive system, hence slowing down the already deficient supply of nutrition. The lack of natural roughage in our diet is accredited to many health related problems suffered in western society. This can obviously be overcome by changing our diet and taking more natural roughage as found in raw vegetables, whole grains and fruit high in fibre.

A balanced diet may not always be practical, and to balance our nutritional needs, supplements of vitamins, minerals and other nutritional ingredients are necessary for our health.

The normal tablet form of these supplements is in over 90% of the products on the shop shelves of a synthetic origin, of which our body, to varying degrees, is able to absorb - usually less than 10%. (The addition of bioflavonoids or chelation to synthetic nutrients increases intake by a small percentage.)

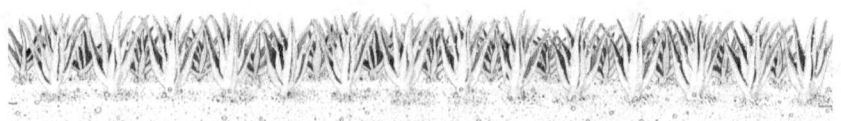

In the past 70 years, on average the nutrition in our foods has decreased by up to 70%.. This is in our modern lifestyle and expenditure, often a problem. To overcome this deficiency we can either find a source of food state supplements, such as those based on herbs, or food state cultivated supplements.

Another good source of obtaining our daily nutritional needs is food state nutritional drinks. Look for a drink which clearly indicates its ability to provide a complete balance of nutrition. There are plenty on the market now days.

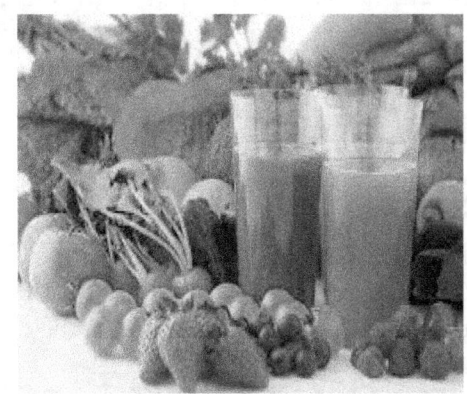

There are also blenders and juicers available to blend and juice fresh fruit and vegetables. These all provide a delicious way of obtaining our sources of nutrition.

By "food state" we refer to ingredients containing the required supplements, which are as found naturally in organic matter, such as vegetables, grains, nuts and fruit; which our digestive system is readily able to utilise.

It has the ability to cleans the digestive system, thus enabling the nutrition available from our food and supplementation to be better absorbed. Hence it is a good idea to take our daily oral supplementation of the Aloe Vera Gel about a half hour or so before taking any food or supplements and meals.

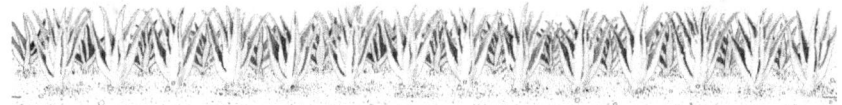

It aids in natural healing which, with its anti-inflammatory abilities, increases the absorption of nutrition.

Its contents of nutritional ingredients would not in the normal understanding of nutrition be anywhere near enough to provide the needs of our body, no matter what quantity we were reasonably expected to take. However, the synergistic effect of its constituent parts, which include biological active body switches can activate the use of the nutrition it does contain, and that otherwise absorbed by the body. Hence it enhances the body's own ability to cope with the environment, degeneration due to ageing, accidental damage or inherited weakness. Taking your oral dose of |Aloe Vera about a half hour before you eat is one of the best ways of enhancing the nutrition you can gain from your diet.

In fact, whichever natural based therapy or even drug therapy a practitioner follows, Aloe Vera Gel will, by its natural built - in abilities, enhance the specialist treatments on offer.

Used on its own, it also has been shown to improve the health of even people who claimed to be in reasonably good health for their age, giving an invigoration and more youthful appearance to those who use it regularly over a period of time both orally and topically.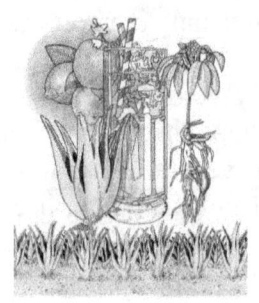

Furthermore, its natural antioxidants and other attributed activities will help protect the body against degenerative diseases such as those mentioned in the above chapters.

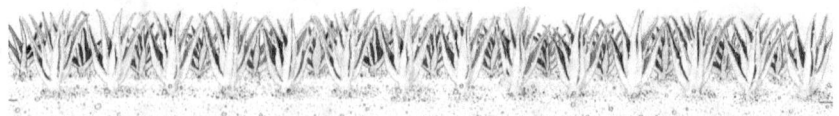

Oral use of Aloe Vera

Dependent on the state of our metabolism, there can sometimes be dormant enzymes in our system which take three months or more to kick into action.

It is therefore advisable to think along the lines of using Aloe Vera Gel for three months or more before expecting positive results in areas of especially degenerative problems. However, I have not yet come across anyone who using the amount I have suggested, has not within three months obtained some positive result from its use.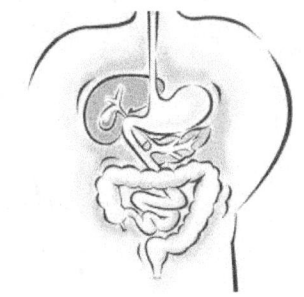

Positive side - effects which have been reported to me are an increase in hair growth and quality, strengthening of the nails, sleeping better, having more energy, becoming more alert, faster reflexes, fewer colds and flu and so on. Generally there is an improvement of the body's overall health.

During that three months you would expect to use at least 5 Ltr. of a 100% stabilised Aloe Vera Gel. We normally advise users to take at least 50 ml a day, which means that a 1 Ltr. bottle would last for 20 days. People with serious problems, who wish to get results quickly can safely use up to 150 ml a day taken as three doses, one before each meal.

With Aloe, the more you take,
the quicker you take it,
the faster the results will come.

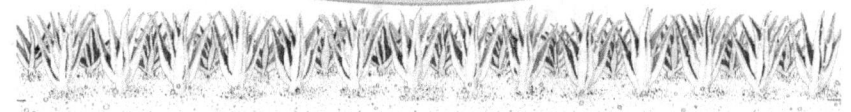

If 50 ml of Aloe has an unpleasant effect due to its potent detoxing activities, lessen the dose as follows. 10 ml days 1 to 3, 20 ml on days 4 to 7, 30 ml teach day of the second week and up to 50 ml thereafter.

**Whoever you are,
or whatever your age,
Aloe Vera Gel has the ability to
increase your state
of well being.**

Uses Today

The following is a sample of information showing in a practical manner from real life situations, what Aloe Vera is being used for and how it is being applied. We in no way make any medical claims on its behalf, simply pass onto you information that is widely available from other source material. If you are concerned by your health, you should consult a either a medical doctor or trained practitioner.

Allergies and other external sources of irritation. As a pain inhibitor, Aloe Vera Gel greatly reduces the problem of itching. It appears to enhance the healing of rashes and sores.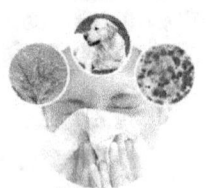

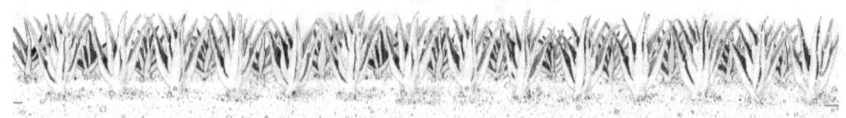

Stings and bites of most types seem to be reduced by its use when applied topically. The internal consumption of the gel seems to speed up this action.

Acne. psoriasis. rashes

Aloe Vera Gel, or Gelly has been applied to the infected areas several times each day. Results indicate that it reduces infection, cleanses the spots and reduces scarring.

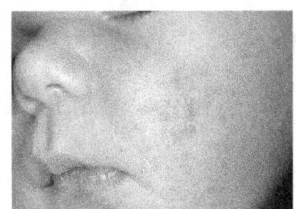

Each person seems to respond differently to its use, some showing signs of improvement within days, while others need weeks of continual use before appearances improve. The internal consumption of Aloe Vera Gel would seem to hasten results. Before topical application is made, thorough cleansing of the infected area with pure soap and water, or lemon or lime juice is recommended. With psoriasis conditions some people find that a 70 - 30 mix of Aloe Gel and cold pressed virgin olive oil is beneficial. The internal use as well as topical application is recommended, as such conditions are thought to be internal as well as external.

Aloe Vera as a Health Drink.

Many people continue using Aloe Vera as a dietary supplement, to maintain maximum health. Aloe Vera Gel is a vegetable juice, and once the seal of the bottle is opened it is best stored in a cool place, or fridge. Taken on an empty stomach, the Gel seems to work best.

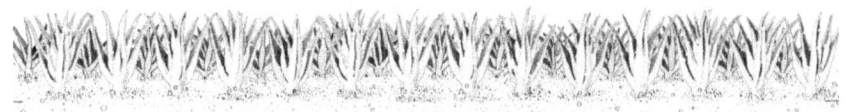

Many users take between 20 and 50 ml a half hour before each meal, or all at once first thing in the morning.

Some people need to take the Aloe Vera Gel for a longer period. Much depends on the following factors:-

Age.

+ The more Aloe Vera Gel we use, the quicker we use it, the faster it can work.

+ Length of time one has had a problem.

+ One's metabolism.

+ General state of health.

+ Stress levels in ones life.

+ Diet.

+ The amount of daily intake of Aloe Vera Gel.

+ The purity of the product being used.

Tests would appear to indicate that the regular use of Aloe Vera helps detoxification from the body of harmful substances, some of which the human body would otherwise be unable to cope with.

With the increase over recent years of man - made pesticides and fertilisers, along with the many E's added to food - and blamed for

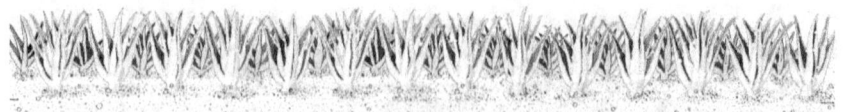

hyperactivity among other things - the use of Aloe Vera Gel as a food supplement would appear to be a good idea.

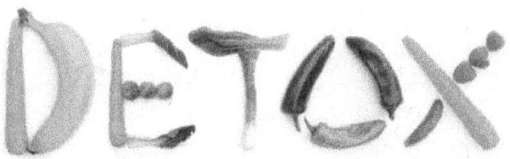

On rare occasions using Aloe Gel internally has been known to bring out the toxins through the skin, causing a slight rash. This usually passes within a few days, and is proof that it is working. If it persists it has been found that lessening the amount you are taking to start with, then gradually building up to higher doses will work better.

To start with, urine is sometimes noticed to be stronger, and stools larger, yet softer. All this is added proof that our body is responding well to the naturalising of our metabolism. Try not to use tea, coffee or alcohol within an hour or so of taking the Gel. Aloe Vera Gel is a hydrator, while these dehydrate and will counter the good Aloe Vera can do.

Arthritis
Many thousands of people who have been drinking an amount of Gel to give between 40 and 60 ml of a 1:1 stabilised Aloe Vera Gel regularly each day claim that their arthritis and other inflammatory conditions, pains them less than it did before. In fact many claim complete freedom from the complaint while using it. It would appear that when it is taken two or three times a day, better results are obtained. Some people find some relief after only

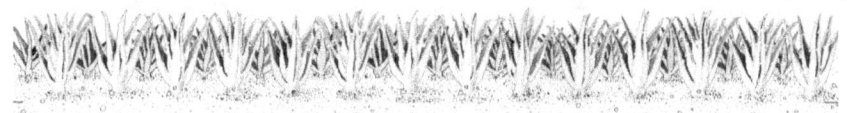

a day or two. Others find that they have to persist with treatment for three to six months or more before relief is felt.

Asthma

The use of orally ingested 100% stabilised Aloe Vera Gel has been used regularly. Two other methods have also been used. Placing some Aloe Gel into boiling water and breathing in the vapour, or placing Aloe Gel into an atomiser. The latter is popular as many asthmatics find it difficult to breathe in steam.

Brown Skin Spots

Brown skin spots which tend to develop at a mature age on areas which have been open to the sun, appear to respond to regular applications of Aloe Gel or Gelly, when used daily over a period of months. The more frequent the application, the faster the result.

Burns and Scalds

Burns are described in four categories:-

1. First degree - skin not broken.

2. Second degree - blisters and skin broken.

3. Third degree - all layers of skin destroyed and wound open.

4. Fourth degree - skin charred.

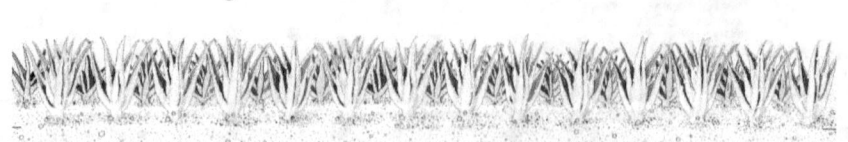

All burns are serious and medical attention is important.

Before application of any medication it is important to have the area thoroughly cleaned from any foreign matter. Aloe Vera Gel applied to burns on a regular basis apparently helps reduce pain, rehydrate the affected area, stop blistering and promote regrowth of new skin, reducing the possibility of infection and scarring.

On first degree burns the Gel or Gelly can be applied in a sterile manner directly to the affected area.

On second degree burns, the gel sprayed onto the area has been found most effective. Reapplication is necessary before the skin dries, until hydration has been achieved. Then three or four times daily to reduce pain and stimulate regrowth.

Aloe Vera has long been attested to for its aid in reducing pain and discomforts associated with sunburn and other burns caused by radiation. The more frequent the application, the speedier the response.

Cuts and Wounds

Documented evidence since the days of Alexander the Great show how effective the Gel of Aloe Vera is in aiding healing of all types of cuts and wounds. The old home remedy is to clean the wound, put Aloe Gel onto it, close it up, bandage and keep the bandage soaked in Aloe Gel. Many attest to the ease of removing bandages, rapid healing, reduction in pain, and little or no scarring when Aloe Vera is used in this way.

Colds and Sinus Conditions

There appear to be three ways in which colds and sinus conditions have been treated with Aloe Gel.

- One manner has been by inhaling vapour containing the gel

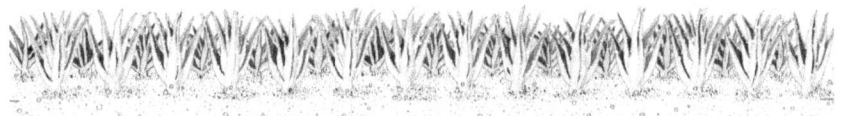

- The other is by taking it internally, to boost the Immune System

- And the final is by spraying the Gel up the nasal passage

Caution for Diabetics

It would appear that over a period of time, the regular use of a 100% stabilised Aloe Vera Gel taken internally, may improve the ability of the pancreas to produce its own insulin. Diabetics are advised to monitor their blood sugar level and according to medical advice, reduce any medication as required to maintain a correct blood sugar level.

Deodorant

Some people, especially those allergic to commercial preparations, have used Aloe Vera Gel or Gelly as a deodorant. It is an historical fact that hunters in Africa from certain tribes have long used Aloe Vera to stop their body odour smell warning the animal of their presence.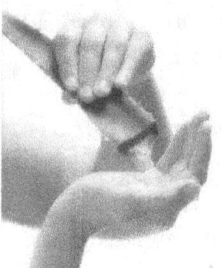

Digestive Problems

Pains in the abdomen may be serious, and consultation of a medical practitioner should be sought. In many parts of the world, where Aloe Grows wild and a medical practitioner is not available, Aloe is the first thing people try. It is often successful, but not always. It appears to balance the system being good for both constipation and dysentery, aiding in digestion, effective in colitis

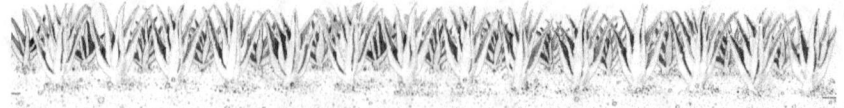

and other inflammations. There are even reports of it helping in cases of kidney infections.

It is worth noting, that although the Gel of the plant helps in cases of constipation, the Gel of itself is not a laxative. It does, however, moisturise the stools. The yellow sap, found between the outer skin and the Gel called aloin is a laxative.

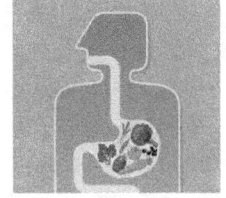

If using the Gel straight from the plant, one should first fillet the gel from the outer leaf, and thoroughly wash away the sap before using.

Earaches

A little Aloe Gel is placed in the ear, and has been used to ease pain and reduce infection. Some people say that warming the gel a little helps.

Eyes

As with the ears, the eye is one of the most delicate organs of the body, and proper medical attention should be given when disorders occur. A few drops of Aloe Vera Gel placed in the eye have been used for centuries. It sometimes stings a little before bringing relief. Sometimes it is mixed 50 / 50 with pure water to reduce the stinging effect.

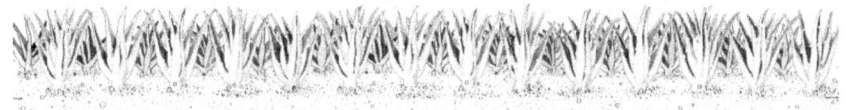

Hair and Scalp

Many shampoos and hair conditioners contain only small amounts of Aloe Vera. A report in the International Journal of Dermatology stated that diseases of the scalp respond very well to the direct application of a 100% stabilised Aloe Vera Gel to the infected areas. Aloe Vera has long been used as a natural shampoo, hair set and conditioner. Remember that Aloe Vera has a drying effect and mixing it with pure pressed olive or rapeseed oil helps avoid this drying effect.

Haemorrhoids

Testimonies indicate a very fast relief from this irritable condition, when the Gel is applied direct to the affected area. In the past a piece of the gel from the leaf would be frozen to give rigidity and then slid into position. Today, however, with the development of Aloe Vera Gelly or ointments, it can be applied directly by use of a swab, cotton wool or tissue, usually after a motion is passed, or after a bath, and as often as it is felt prudent.

Infections

Medical reports down through the ages to our modern times stress the lack of infection when Aloe Vera is used on open wounds, abrasions and cuts. The leaf was split open and the gel side of the leaf placed directly on the affected area, acting as a bandage and carrier of the healing gel. Today lotions and Gelly are available for convenient use.

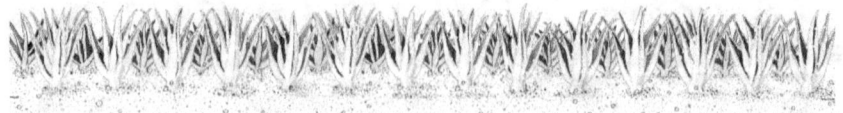

Insect Repellent

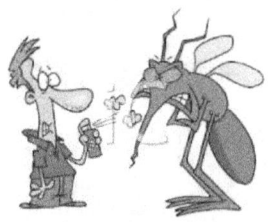

Aloe Gel rubbed on the skin has long been used as an insect repellent. In the West Indies it is often used in delousing animals.

Mouthwash sore throats and mouth ulcers

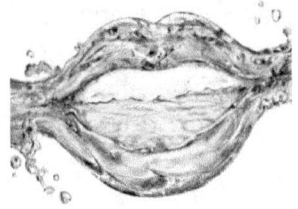

The Gel can be diluted, gargled with or drunk and will help in eliminating germs or bad breath. Mouth ulcers often react favourably to repeated swilling of the Gel over the affected area.

Scar Removal

As already indicated, many people testify that frequent and regular use of Aloe Vera Gel on the affected area may help in reducing scars. The older the scar, the longer it seems to take.

Stretch Marks

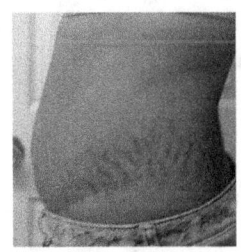

Many women who know of the benefits, use Aloe Vera over the abdomen to aid the skin in adjusting to the stresses of pregnancy. After delivery they continue using it to help in the contraction of skin

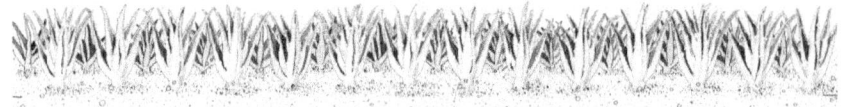

mass and to lessen the stretch marks so often left behind. It is widely used on areas when weight loss has occurred as it can help eliminate surplus skin.

Ulcers

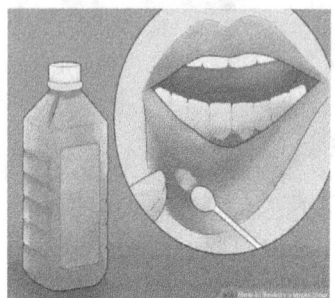

A very serious condition, ulcerations should always be given medical attention. Aloe Vera applied to the affected area has been shown in many tests to be a very effective treatment. Both topical application, by soaking the applied sterile bandage etc., and internal drinking of the Gel.

Varicose Veins

Obviously this serious condition should receive medical attention. Many people have used Aloe Vera on the affected areas to varying degrees of satisfaction. The internal use of the Gel, as well as topical application, seems to enhance the positive results.

The above demonstrates how many users are today using Aloe Vera. Although your complaint may not be mentioned, from the above you should have a good idea of how to use this completely safe product.

Aloe Vera is after all just a vegetable, related to the onion and garlic family of plants.

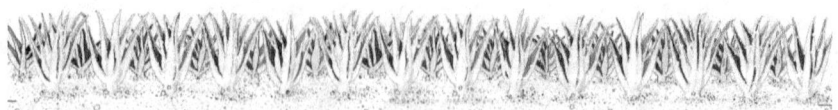

Does Aloe Vera have Side Effects?

In a test conducted by Dr Jeffrey Bland of the Linus Pauling Institute of Science and Medicine in California in 1985, one person in 10 noticed a slight digestive gas problem, which diminished after daily use over a week.

Dr Peter Atherton personally known by the author stated that most reactions to Aloe Vera products was due to the other substances added to the product.

Dr Atherton quotes Guy's hospital in London as saying that ingestion of Whole Leaf Aloe had in a few cases resulted in abdominal pains and diarrhea.

What the Doctors Say

I have often been asked, as I queried when first introduced to Aloe Vera, "Why don't doctors use it"?

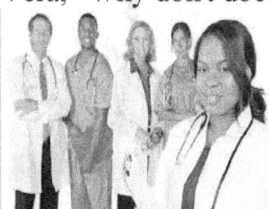 The answer is that there are doctors who do use it. In fact, those that have researched the subject use it regularly. However, in the closed shop situation operated by the doctors union, the BMA in the U. K., and taking into account the fields in which doctors have been trained, medical staff naturally turn to the products manufactured by the pharmaceutical industry.

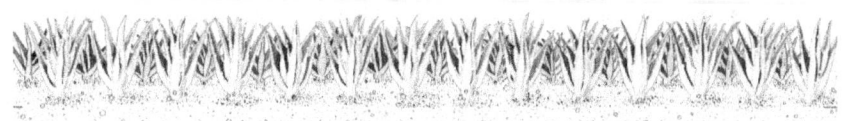

As already mentioned, no matter how good Aloe Vera Gel is, no pharmaceutical company can afford to licence a product which is not going to earn them a return on their financial outlay. Hence the medical periodicals sent to the doctors, as a rule do not contain information about Aloe Vera.

On the other hand the natural healing practitioner believes in aiding and strengthening the process of the body, whether that be by stimulation, such as by way of:-

- ✓ Acupuncture,
- ✓ Homeopathy,
- ✓ Medical Massage,
- ✓ Nutrition.
- ✓ Biological Activities of Aloe Vera Gel,

It is my judgement that all fields of medicine need to work together for the benefit of mankind, and am pleased that this view is endorsed by members of the royal family, and a growing number of medical specialists.

1 Acute injury to muscles - joints - tendons - and arthritis:

The treatment used was Aloe Vera Gelly, and Aloe Vera Liniment, often called Aloe Vera Rub, applied topically; and Aloe Vera Gel taken orally.
The results were as follows:-

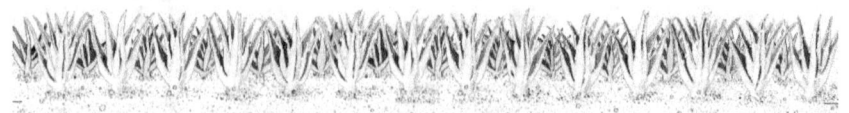

- Penetration ... superior to other products.

- Reduction of swelling ... good and usually superior to other products.

- Relief of pain ... superior to other products.

- Anti-inflammatory ... superior to other products.

- Improved mobility ... good and sometimes superior to other products.

- Healing acceleration ... superior to other products.

- Antiseptic ... superior on abrasions, contusions and lacerations, otherwise about the same as other products.

2 The treatment of burns

In the treatment of thermal, radiation and chemical bums, using the Aloe Vera Gel, Gelly, Lotion or ointment - the results were superior to all other products available, as:-

- a pain reliever ...

- anti-inflammatory ...

- blister inhibitor ...

- healing acceleration ...

- anti-puritic ... and penetration.

- As an antiseptic it proved to be equal to other products.

- In the treatment of thermal burns, its moisturising effect was also superior to that of other products available.

3 Infections
including, decubitous ulcers, leg ulcers, radiation ulcers, impetigo, tonsillitis, fever blisters, candida albicans, vaginitis, cervicitis dermatitis, acne vulgaris, herpes simplex, contact dermatitis, eczema, haemorrhoids, liver spots, gingivectomy, open wound surgery, tinea and warts.

Aloe Vera used in treatments of these problems were superior in relief of pain, penetration and acceleration of healing.

4 Allergies
Allergic conditions such as skin problems, insect bites and stings, eczema and contact dermatitis.

Aloe Vera was found good in relief of:-

- pain,
- reducing swelling,
- in penetration,
- healing,
- anti-inflammatory agent,
- anti pruritic
- anti endemic.

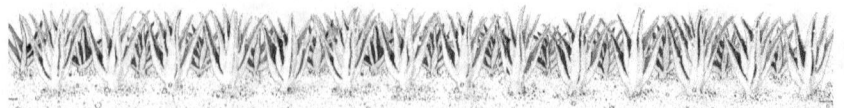

More detailed analytical results of clinical tests from which these abbreviated notes are taken can be found in the "Silent Healer" and "Healing Winners" by B. C. Coates Ph.D.

5 HIV

"Aloe is to an AIDS patient such as insulin is to a diabetic".
Terry L. Pulse, M. D.

In 1981 the HIV virus was first identified. Since its onset the pharmaceutical industry and laboratories around the world have been busy trying to find a cure to this possible plague. Dr. Terry Pulse and Dr. Robert B. Strecker MD, have both conducted clinical tests on AIDS patients, with varying degrees of immune deficiency, at various stages of the infection. At all stages, oral application of Aloe Vera Gel given a minimum of 400 ml of the pure Aloe Gel a day, has given positive results.

A pilot study conducted in 1990 on 29 AIDS patients, resulted with a substantial number of patients physically improving. Energy levels improved, fever disappeared, night sweats stopped, cough decreased or stopped, shortness of breath decreased, lymph nodes decreased in size, diarrhoea stopped, weakness improved. Hypersensitivity skin tests improved. In 96.4% of tested patients, their modified Walter Reed scores were improved at 180 days. Kamofsky scores improved in 93.1 %. T4 lymphaticytes increased, and in some their reactive HIV P24 antigen converted to negative. In effect, Aloe Vera Gel showed itself to be a far more impressive agent for countering AIDS than other recognised medication.
Information from the ",Journal of Advancement in Medicine" Winter 1990.
Quoted in "Aloe Vera A Mission Discovered" by Dr. Lee Ritter.

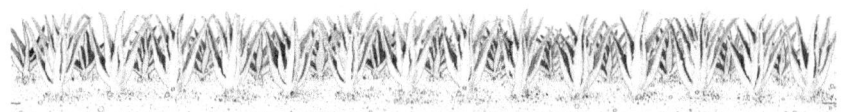

6   Dr. Peter Atherton MB ChB. D.Obst. R.C.O.G. M.R.C.G.P., an NHS doctor practising in Buckinghamshire, was until recently a staunch supporter of only orthodox medicine. He researched the plant and found to his astonishment that 39 out of the 40 research papers he studied were positive, a higher rating than many accepted drugs now on the market. At the time of writing this book, he is further researching the subject of Aloe Vera at Oxford University.
Quoted from "Daily Mail 14/2/1995" by Hazel Courtney.

7   Dr. Greg Henderson another specialist, and head of a multi - practice clinic in America, claims that tests on Aloe Vera have also shown that it is a natural "Anti-inflammatory" a "Growth Stimulator" and a "Detoxifier". He concludes by saying that if you absorb Aloe Vera you get increased regeneration. Once your regeneration process is increased then you get better absorption of nutrition and body function, which leads to better assimilation or processing. Giving better nutrition and more energy - that quality of life you cannot get in any other way than when the body is functioning normally.

Testimonies.

In this chapter we have the opportunity to explore some of the many testimonies of users known to the author.

Birmingham.
A family friend, 92 years young at the time was crippled with arthritis. Her mobility was seriously impaired she being able to move only with the aid of her walking sticks. Her hands were

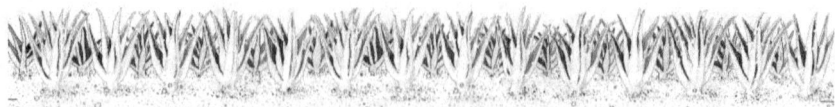

misshapen and she was no longer able to play her piano. As a life long pianist and teacher of music, she felt this disability badly. She couldn't bear to be parted from her old piano, and swore that she would be able to play it again one day. Her face was covered with brown skin spots, which with the wrinkles made her look her age.

On hearing of the success of others with the regular use of Aloe Gel, she decided to try it for herself. I called at her house about two weeks later, confidently expecting her to be proclaiming the joys of this wonder of nature. Upon asking her how she felt, she answered, "About the same as usual". Then all of a sudden she got up out of her chair, walked straight to the back door, and chased a dog out of her garden, Came back in and sat down. I was amazed at how freely she had moved, and looking around the room couldn't see her walking sticks. So I asked her where they were. "Oh" she exclaimed, "I don't know, maybe they are in the front room. I haven't used them for a couple of days."

Now I felt better, for I could see how Aloe Vera was working. Slowly and surely without noticeable side effects.

It was nearly six months before I called by again. I rang the door bell and was pleased to see a lady which at first glance I took to be her daughter come to the door. What a change, gone were the brown skin spots and wrinkles. She even took me to the piano I had repaired for her, and played if for me. "There," she boasted, I told you I would play again. See my hands are normal again. The swellings and stiffness are gone.

Yes, you guessed it. She had continued using the Aloe Vera Gel regularly, three times a day. She also kept a saucer with some in it, to dip her fingers into and pat over her face regularly, at least three or four times a day. You can guess that I walked out of her house that day on air. It is experiences like that which motivate me to share with you the joy that Aloe can bring.

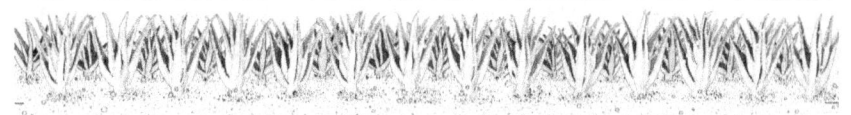

E. B. Birmingham.
My son introduced me to Aloe Vera, persuading me to use a wine glass a day of the Aloe Gel for my arthritis. This I did, and although sceptical to begin with, I found that after only a few days the pains I had suffered with for years had eased. In fact, my wrist which had been particularly bad was completely free of pain within only a week. I also found an improvement in my sciatica. Continued use of Aloe Vera has even helped my angina, which has just disappeared from my life. A welcome departure. I am going to continue using Aloe Vera for the remainder of my life.

W. G. B. RMN. SEN. Birmingham.
My heart literally stopped three times. I had some five hours earlier eaten some contaminated corned beef in a sandwich obtained at work. Shortly after this I started vomiting and pushed just about everything out of my stomach from both ends, to the point of rupturing the stomach lining and damaging the duodenum. A nurse friend of our family resuscitated me three times while we waited for the ambulance to arrive. After this I had to learn to live with a very painful duodenal ulcer, which seemed to ebb and flow from time to time. I was going through one of the painful periods when my mother gave me some Aloe Vera Gel. Naturally, my nurse's training told me to beware of these "Jungle Juices", these "Elixiers of Youth", which I took to be mere folk law. So in the fridge it went, and on with the pain for a couple more weeks, until my brother, who had no medical training whatever came to see me. His first comment was: "You haven't used any of the Aloe Gel have you?" How could he know that, unless this juice really does work. He then told me of how it had helped his stomach ulcer, how he was eating chips and things I couldn't even dream of. So reasoning that a Herb couldn't do me any harm, and being in pain in the early hours one morning, I poured out half a pint and drank

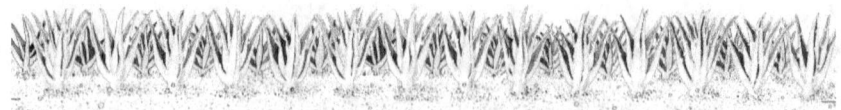

it down quickly. To my surprise I felt something happen inside my stomach within moments of doing so. Something was moving. Wind passed, motions eased and pain decreased within days of starting to regularly drink this juice. Today I no longer take the 50 or so tablets I had been on, nor do have to be so careful about my diet. My allergies which I was injecting myself for every three days disappeared after six weeks. The pain from the damage I did to my back whilst nursing has also cleared up. Working on my car, I burned myself on the manifold, so on went the Aloe Vera Gelly, away went the pain, and now I share Aloe Vera with others myself. I highly recommend its use to anyone.

G. M. Birmingham.

We were building a small greenhouse in my mother's back yard, when some creosote splashed into her eye. It was swollen up badly, looked very bloodshot and irritated badly. She washed it with eyewash, but was still in a bad way. I suggested straining some Aloe Vera Gel and using that as an eyewash. She did so, and within an hour the swelling had gone down. Yes, it stung her to start with, but within a minute or so the irritation, the pain and the swelling had gone.

On another occasion, while working in her garden, a wasp stung the back of her hand, which immediately swelled up badly. She took a drink of the Aloe Vera Gel and applied some to the sting itself. Within a few minutes the pain was gone and a couple of hours later the swelling had disappeared.

M. G. London.

One day, working on stage setting up the lights for a musical, I sliced off a chunk of my index finger with the lens of one of the stage lights I was carrying. Blood was everywhere. Looking at this hole in my finger I could see the bone, and hanging from it the

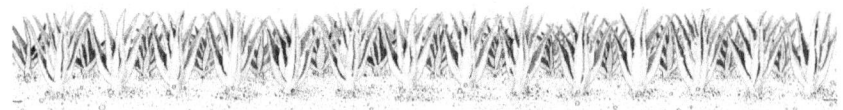

chunk of flesh that had been the tip of my finger. Out came my first aid tube of Aloe Vera Gelly. I squeezed some into the hole, replaced the flesh and bandaged the finger. Within minutes the throbbing has gone, bleeding had stopped and I was working again. Phew, I thought later, am I glad for that Gelly. The amazing fact is that two days later when I removed the bandage, the skin had knit back into place with very little scarring.

E. B. Birmingham.

My son had occasionally developed a sty in his eye. It usually lasted for three to four days before doctor's medication would help It clear up. Having some Aloe Vera Gel handy, I strained some and used that in the eye instead. We applied it by way of a cotton swab, slowly letting it penetrate into the eye, so as not to irritate the youngster too much. Within three hours of this one application, all signs of the sty had disappeared. It has never recurred since, thanks to Aloe.

G. M. Birmingham.

My wife had always suffered with a lack of iron when carrying our children. However, with our last daughter she was using a wine glass of Aloe Vera Gel each day. She never once had to use iron tablets, nor did she suffer with morning sickness or other maladies throughout her pregnancy. She also found that it eased her monthly problems too.

Ms. A. Birmingham.

Our friend was so stiff and overweight, she could hardly walk down the street. One day, seeing me up to my arms in muck, gardening, she commented on how well I looked. So I told her of how Aloe Vera Gel had helped me. She knew it as "Sinkle Bible"

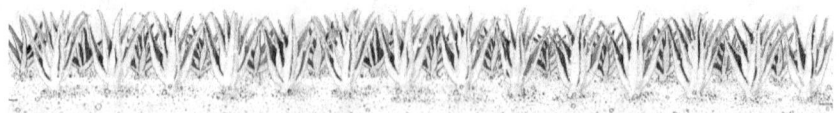

from her native Jamaica. So she started using it, a small glass a day the first week, two glasses a day the second week. By the end of the third week she was feeling so much better that there was a definite spring in her step. She did a knees up mother brown just to demonstrate to us how much better she was feeling. Her blood pressure problems, arthritis and diabetes had all improved to the point of being taken off of some of the medication by her doctor. That summer she was climbing ladders redecorating her house.

D. B. Gloucester.
When first told about Aloe Vera, my wife, a nurse, and I were most sceptical. However, having been persuaded into obtaining a bottle, I thought I might as well use it. To my amazement, although I had always thought myself in good health, my general well - being had got up and got better. No longer did I feel so tired after a long day's work. My athlete's foot had all but run away. Today I share the joys of this jungle juice with others, and see them join in a brighter life with me.

Z. B. Gloucester.
I have suffered with muscular contractions for 20 years. The doctors told me there was nothing they could do for me. Within three months of using a wine glass of Aloe Vera Gel each day, the contractions had completely stopped

L. B. Wolverhampton.
Using Aloe Vera Gelly for just three days completely cleared up my chilblains, which I had suffered with for nearly 20 years.

C. I. Gloucester.
For a period of three years or so I suffered with migraine headaches. The doctors and specialists could find nothing wrong

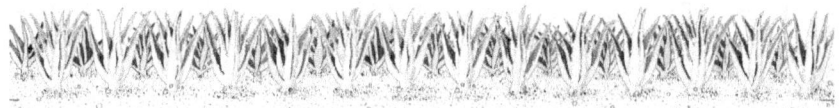

with me. When I was introduced to Aloe Vera, and started using it for myself, I found that these headaches just went away. They have not recurred since first starting to take Aloe Vera Juice.

l. J. Gloucester.
For 16 years I have suffered with hayfever. The doctor's tablets didn't completely control it, the tablets just made me sleepy. After using Aloe Vera for six months, my hayfever has completely stopped. Today I feel much better.

P. B. Gloucester
Before using Aloe Vera I had continually suffered with colds and flu. Today, after using Aloe Vera as part of my daily diet, I have found a general improvement in my well being. Colds and flu seem to be keeping clear of me. Maybe the germs don't like its bitter taste!

R. P. Walsall.
For 20 years of my 82 - year life I have been housebound with leg ulcers. In fact I had to give up my nursing career because of them. At times doctors had thought that amputation was the only answer. However I pressed on using good nursing, massage and, with persistence, struggled through.
Other problems started to creep up on me over the years. Varicose eczema, lymphatic blockage of the ankle a peptic stomach ulcer, rheumatism, arthritis and a chest infection that just would not go away, bowel troubles and retention of urine. I have so far taken over a three - week period, two litres of a ready to drink Aloe Vera Gel, and a tube of Aloe Vera Gelly topically on the leg ulcers. I now have no pain or sign of the chest infection. The rheumatic and arthritic pains have greatly lessened, and my appetite has improved. My stomach disorders appear to be righting themselves.

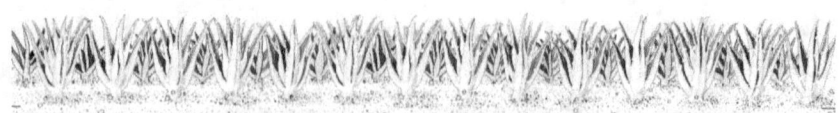

The leg ulcer is the most dramatic; it has been reduced from the size of a man's fist to just a small mark on the leg. The first couple of days, when changing the dressing, lots of muck came away from the ulceration, leaving after it nice clean flesh, which rapidly healed. I am no longer a prisoner in my own home, thanks to Aloe Vera.

Questions I am often asked.

Will Aloe Vera cure my problems?

Only your body can cure your problem.
Aloe Vera can be of benefit even to the fittest person, balancing the metabolism and aiding the natural processes of the body. I have seldom come across anyone who has not responded positively to the persistent use of the Aloe Vera Gel, when taken in sufficient quantities over a period of three months or more of daily use. Aloe Vera Gel appears able to enable your body to do its job as it is meant to.

How do I know which Aloe Vera Juice or Gel to use?

I refer you to the chapter on the subject. But in brief, use a 100% stabilised Aloe Vera Gel in preference the weaker juices available.

How much Aloe Vera Gel should I take?

Every person's needs vary. You are different to everyone else. Therefore your needs could be different to mine. However, as Aloe Vera gel is just a natural vegetable juice, it is as safe to use as apple, orange or carrot juice. Many people continue using Aloe Vera as a dietary supplement, to maintain maximum health.

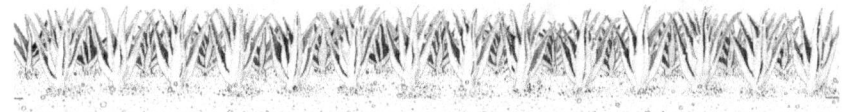

Aloe Vera Gel is a vegetable juice, and once the seal of the bottle is opened, it is best stored in a cool place, or fridge. Taken on an empty stomach the Gel seems to work best. Many users take about 50ml a half hour before each meal to start with, for at least three months. Some doctors I know of prescribe up to 150ml a day of the pure natural Aloe Gel. As drinks containing alcohol is dehydrating, it works against the natural processes of the body. Caffeine also works against the natural processes of the body. Users are advised not to take such drinks within a few hours of using nutritional supplements such as the Aloe Vera Gel. Most users have found that after about three months / 90 days they obtain a positive effect; and are able to lessen the daily amount they take, dependent on their metabolism. I now use about 50 ml a day to help maintain my health. Be patient as some of the amino acids in the Gel take up to three months before they start working in the human body. Children and animals appear to react faster than we adults.

Is Aloe Vera safe to take with other medicines, drugs or herbs?

Throughout all the years my family and I have been involved with the use of Aloe Vera, we have not found one instance where Aloe Vera has had a negative effect upon the effects of a drug or herb. In fact, usually the opposite is true. Aloe Vera appears in practice to enhance the beneficial effects of drugs and herbs, while lessening the side effects of drugs. If you have diabetes or high blood pressure, because the beneficial effects of Aloe will create rapid changes we would recommend the following.
Diabetics. Watch your blood sugar level, and in accordance with your general practitioner's instructions, vary your insulin intake as required.

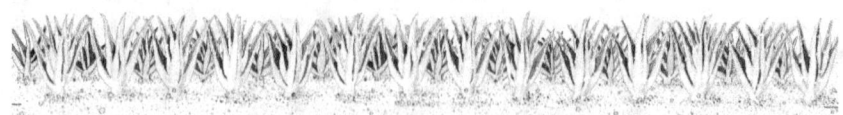

High blood pressure. Start with a smaller dose of just 10 ml, increasing as your body allows, without causing fluctuations, until you reach 100 ml a day. The detoxifying effect of Aloe Vera Gel can sometimes be felt. Dehydration is a major cause of medical problems. Through ill health, ageing, disease, inherited weakness, or accident, a lack of enough pure water each day, use of caffeine and alcohol, stress, electricity, chemical and other pollution; the body creates cholesterol to protect the individual cells which hinders the flow of liquid in and out of them. In this state it is unable to use vitamin B6, which affects the utilisation of the minerals, magnesium, and zinc. Also the work of amino acids such as tryptophan, taurine and methionine are also negated. Toxicity within the cells builds up, slowing down their natural functions. ALOE VERA GEL contains 95% water, which acts as though it has a lower surface tension than normal water and has the ability to strip the cells of cholesterol, thus force liquids carrying nutrients into the cells, and toxins out of them. This creates a natural flow within the body, and enables cells within the glands, organs and muscle tissue to operate to their optimum. Hence normal health is induced.

I am a diabetic. Can I take Aloe Vera?

Many diabetics do so, and have found that their dependence on taking insulin and tablets can lessen. In some cases I know of, it has been totally eliminated. It is therefore advisable that you keep a close watch on your blood sugars.

Can I take other vitamin and mineral supplements with Aloe Vera?

Yes indeed you can. In fact many users claim that other products work better when taking the Gel.

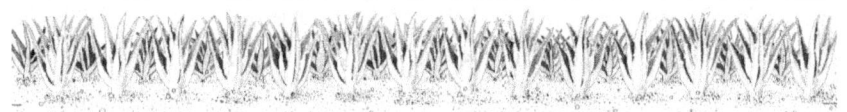

Is it worth my while using Aloe Vera Gel if I feel fit?

Yes, other such people have found that they become more resistant to colds and flu, and have greater energy levels while taking the Gel.

Does the pure Aloe Vera Gel colour and taste vary?

Yes it can, according to season and the amount of rainfall. In fact beware of products that don't. Just as the taste of one orange or apple varies compared with another, so can the Gel from the Aloe plant. In fact if your product doesn't vary in colour and taste it is because it has been so highly processed that its biological therapeutic abilities would be suspect.

Will using Aloe Vera affect the drugs my doctor is giving me?

According to professional advice and personal experience, there are no known adverse reactions. In fact, I have personally noticed that side effects from drugs lessen, and the beneficial effects are enhanced while taking the Gel.

Can a baby take Aloe Vera to drink?

My family and other users have used Aloe Vera Gel with all our baby's since they were old enough to take solid food. In all our research we have not found any reports of harmful side effects to any user, baby or adult.
However, one doctor recently involved in the use of Aloe Vera suggested waiting for a child's digestive system to fully develop before ingesting. He suggests waiting for a child to reach 18 months of age.

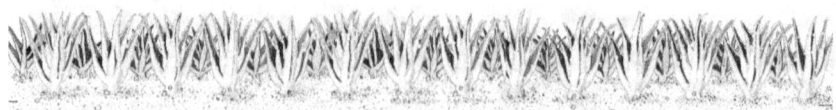

References and research papers.

The following chapter is a list of research papers, from which all the scientific information contained in this publication has originated.

In the past three years alone, nearly 400 more papers on the use of Aloe Vera are reported to have been created.

The scientific interest in the biological activities of this one plant has grown at an astonishing rate. Such has been the astonishing results of experiments, that medical researchers at Oxford, England among many other centres are being converted. The following pages speak for themselves.

We have recorded them in the following order:-

The name of the main researcher.

The year the research was first reported.

The name of the research paper or book.

In the case of research papers, the name of the journal it was published in, with page and chapter references, or place of publication.

Abraham
1979   Occurrence of triploidy in Aloe Vera Tourn   Current Science 48:1001-1002

Afzal
1991   Identification of some prostanoids in Aloe Vera extractsPlanta Medica. 1991. 57(1). 38 - 40.

Agarwal
1985   Prevention of atheromatous heart disease   Angiology 1985. 36(8) 485 - 492.

Ahmad
1993   A biologically active and potential medicinal plant   Hambard 1993. 36(1). 108 - 115.

Ajabmoor
1990   Effects of Aloes on blood glucose levels .... Ethnopharmacology. 1990. Feb. 28.(2). 215 - 220.

Aleshkini
1957   An Aloe emulsion   USSR 11:54-55

Anderson
1983   Aloe Vera Juice: A Veterinary predicament? 5: S364-S368

Anderson
1991   In vitro veridical activity of selected anthraquinones.... Antiviral Res. 1991. Sep. 16(2). 185 - 196.

Anon

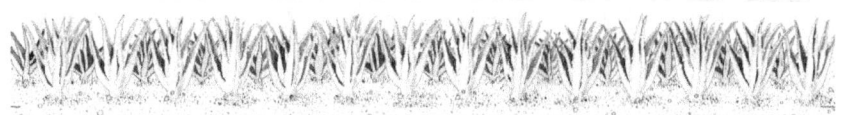

1977   A. V. The Ageless Botanical   Soap, Cosmetic, Chemical
     Specialities 53: 34-38
Anon
1980   British Pharmacopoeia   HMSO. London
Anon
1981   Moisturiser efficacy measured quantitatively using electrical conductivity
     parameter   F. D. C. reports 2, 5.
Anton
1980   Therapeutical use of natural anthraquinones....   Pharmacology 20
     (suppl. 1) 104-112
Ashleye
1957   Aloe Vera in the treatment of thermal and irradiation burns Plastic and
     Reconstructive Surgery. 20: 383-396
Ashleye
1993   Applying heat during processing Aloe Vera Gel   Erde
     International. 1:40-44
Atherton
1997   The Essential Aloe Vera.
Bader
1981   Natural hydroxyanthracenic polyglycosides as sun screens
          Cosmetic & Toiletries 96:67-74
Banks
Natures Genie
Barnes
1947   The healing action of extracts of Aloe leaf of abrasions of the human
     skin American Journal of Botany 34:597
Batchelder
1964   Aloe Vera Herbarist   30:25-29
Beaumont
1964   Homonataloin in Aloe species   Planta Medica   50:505-508
Benigni
1950   Substances with antibiotic action.... Chem. Ab. 1950. 44. 11036.
Beppu
1991   Hypoglycaemic and anti-diabetic effects of Aloe.....   int. Cong. of
     Phytotherapy. Oct. Seoul. Korea. 44.
Beppu
1991   Isolation & the pharmacological activities of the effective compounds
     Aloe .....   International Congress of Phytotherapy. Oct. Seol, korea. 37.
Beppu
1993   Hypoglycaemic and anti-diabetic effects of Aloe.....Phytotherapy
     research 7. 837 - 842.
Bishop

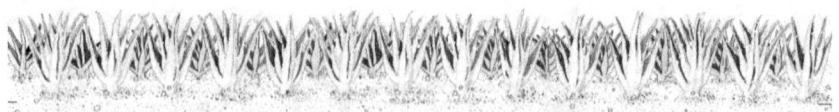

1992   A prospective randomised evaluation - blinded trial of two potential wound healing agents for the treatment of venous stasis ulcers.   J. Vasc. Surg. 16. 251 - 257.

Bland
Research paper

Bland
1985   Effects of orally consumed A. V. juice on gastrointestinal function in normal humans.   Linus Pauling Institute of Science & Medicine Palo Alto. C. A. Prevention Magazine.

Blitz
1963   Aloe Vera Gel in peptic ulcer therapy   Journal of the American Osteopathic Association 62:731-735

Bloomfield
1985   Miracle Plants   Century. ISBN 0 7126 1007 3

Blouchey
1969   Chemical studies of Aloe Vera Juice   Quarterly Journal of Crude Drug Research 9:1445-1453

Bogs
1966   On the preparation and testing of Aloe extract....   Pharmazie 21:547-550

Bouthet
1995   Stimulation of neuron like cell growth of Aloe substances Phytother research 1995. 9. 185-188

Bovik
1966   Aloe Vera, Panacea or old wives tales   Texas Dental Journal 84:13-16

Bradshaw
1996   A. V. its influence on the physiology of wound healing and inflammation J. Brit. Pod. Med. 1996. 51(2). 25 - 29. A7

Brandham
     1985   Jodrel Laboratory, Royal Botanic Gardens, Kew. Surrey. UK.   Personal communication

Brasher
1969   The effects of prednisolone indomethacin and Aloe Vera on tissue culture cells   Oral Surgery, Oral Medicine & Oral Pathology 27:122-128

Brown
1980   A review of the genetic effects of naturally occuring flavanoids.... Mutat Res. 1980. 75. 243 - 277.

Bruce
1967   Investigations of the antibacterial activity of Aloe   South African Medical Journal 41:984

Bruce
1975   Medicinal Properties in the Aloe   Excelsa 5:57-68

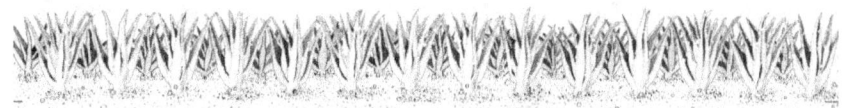

Capasso
1983   Effect of indomethacin on aloin ....   Prostaglandins 26:557-
    562
Carpenter
1991   Clinical applications of a biological response modifier (acemannan) in
    veterinary medicine.   Int. Congress of Phytotherapy. 1991 Oct. Seoul
    Korea. 62.
Cera
1980   The therapeutic efficacy of Aloe Vera cream in thermal injuries Journal
    of the American Animal Hospital Assoc. 16:768-772
Cera
1982   Therapeutic protocol for thermally injured animals ....   Journal
    of the American Animal Hospital Assoc. 18:633-638
Che
1991   Isolation of a human intestinal bacterium capable of transforming
    barbaloin to Aloe emodin anthrone. Planta Med. 1991. Feb. 57(1). 15 - 19.
Cheney
1970   Aloe drug in human therapy   Quarterly Journal of Crudse Drug
    Research 10:1523-1530
Chopra
1956   Glossary of Indian Medicinal plants Council of Scientific and Industrial
    Research. New Dehli
Clumeck
1988   Antiviral drugs other than zidovudine & immun. therapies ... The Am. J.
    of Med. 1988. 85. 165 - 170.
Coats
1979   Silent Healer   P.O. Box. 402 66 Garland Texas
Coats
1981   Healing Winners P.O. Box. 402 66 Garland Texas
Coats
1983   Modern Study of Aloe Vera   P.O. Box. 402 66 Garland Texas

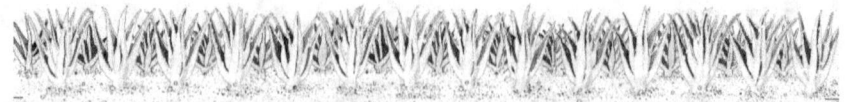

Cole
1943   Aloe Vera in Oriental dermatology   Archives of Dermatology &
    Syphilology 47:250
Collins
1935   Roentgen dermstitis treated with fresh whole leaf od Aloe Vera
    American Journal of Roentgenology 33:396-397
Crewe
1937   The external use of Aloes   Minnesota Medicine 20:670-673
Crewe
1939   Aloes in the treatment of burns and scalds   Minnesota Medicine
    22:538-539
Crosswhite
1984   Aloe Vera, plant symbolism and the threshing floor   Desert plants
    6:43-50
Cutak
1937   Aloe Vera as a remedy for burns   Missouri Botanical Garden Bulletin
    25:169-174
Danhof
1983   Stabilised Aloe Vera - effect on human skin cells   Drug and
    Cosmetic Indutry 1983. 133. 52,54, 105-106
Danhof
1987   Aloe in cosmetics, does it do anything?   Cosmet. Toilet. 1987. 102.
    62 - 63.
Dastur
1962   Aloe Barbadensis Miller   Medicinal Plants of India & Pakistan. pp16-
    17
Davenport
1994   Pharmacists & the silent healer A. V.   Texas Pharmacy. 1994
    July. 113. 18 - 19.
Davis R. H.
1991   Isolation of a stimulatory system in an aloe extract   J Am Podiatr
    Med Ass 81 (9) 473-478
Davis R. H.
1984   Anti-inflammatory and wound healing activity...   J. Am. Podiatric
    Med. Assoc. 1984. Feb. 84.
Davis R. H.
1986   Antiarthretic activity of ... aloe for podiatric medicine.   J. Am. Podiatric
    Med. Assoc. 1986. 76(2) 61-66.
Davis R. H.
1987   Aloe Vera and wound healing.   J. Am. Podiatric Med. Assoc. 1987.
    77(4). 165 - 169.
Davis R. H.

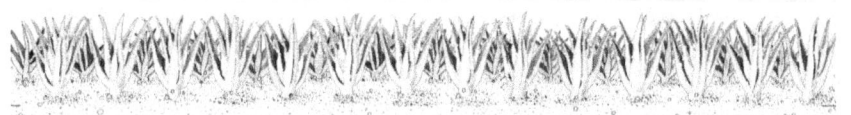

1987   Aloe Vera and inflammations.   Proc. Pa. Acad. Sci. 1986. (recd. 1987) 60(1) 67 - 70.

Davis R. H.
1987   Topical anti-inflammatory activity of A. V. as measured by ear swelling. J. Am. Podiatric Med. Assoc. 1987. 77(11) 610 - 612.

Davis R. H.
1989   Anti inflammatory activity of A. V. against a spectrum of irritants. J. Am. Podiatric Med. Assoc. 1989 June. 79(6) 263 - 276.

Davis R. H.
1988   A natural approach for treating wounds, edema, and pain in diabetes. J. Am. Podiatric |Med. Assoc. 1988. 78(2). 60 - 68.

Davis R. H.
1989   Aloe Vera and gibberellin. Anti inflammatory activities in diabetes. J. Am. Podiatric Med. Assoc. 1989 Jan. 79(1) 24 - 26..

Davis R. H.
1989   Processed A. V. administered topically inhibits inflammation.   J. Am. Podiatric Med. Assoc. 1989 79(8). 395-397..

Davis R. H.
1991   A. V. as a biologically active vehicle for hydrocortisone acetate. J. Am. Podiatric Med. Assoc. 1991. 81(1) 1-9. A3.

Davis R. H.
1991   Influence of Aloe on inflammation and wound healing. International Congress of Phytotherapy 1991. Oct. Seoul. Korea. 29.

Davis R. H.
1992   A. V. and the inflamed synovial pouch model.   J. Am. Podiatric Med. Assoc. 1992. mar. 82(3). 140-148.

Davis R. H.
1993   Biological activity of A. V.   Seigen. Oele. Fette. Wachse (Germany) 1993. sept. 119. 646 - 649.

Davis R. H.
1994   Anti-inflammatory and wound healing activity of a growth substance in A. V. J. Am. Podiatric Med. Assoc. 1994 Feb. 84.(2) 77-81.

Davis R. H.
1994   A.V. hydrocortisone and sterol influence on wound tensile strength and anti-inflammation.   J. Am. Podiatric Med. Assoc. 1994 dec. 84(12). 614-621.

Dixit
1983   Effect of Aloe B. and clofibrate on serum lipids in triton induced hyperlipidaemia in presbytis - entillus - monkey.   Indian. J. Med. Res. 78 (Sept.) 1983. (Recd. 1984). 417 - 421.

Dominguert-Soto
1992   Photodermatitus to A. V.   Int. J.Dermatol. 1992. May. 31(5). 372.

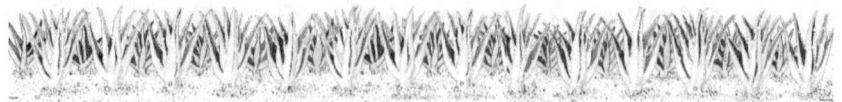

F.D.A.
1982   Russian Sources. parts 170 - 199
Fairbairn1964   The anthracene derivatives of medicinal plants   Lloydia
    27:79-87
Fairbairn
1963   The quantitative conversion of barbaloin to Aloe-Emodin and its
    application to tyhe evaluation of Aloes.   J. of Pharmacy and Pharmacology
    1963. 15.
Farkas
1963   Topical medicament including polyuronide derived from Aloe   US
    patent 3,103,466
Feil
1980   Aloe cosmetics   Bestways (USA) August 1980 p 108
Fine
1959   Cultivation and clinical application of Aloe Vera leaf   Radiology
    31:735-736
Fischer
1982   Medical use of Aloe products   US Pharm. 1982 Aug 7 37 - 45.
Flagg
1959   Aloe Vera gel in dermatological preparations American Perfumer &
    Aromatics 74:27-28, 61
Flesch
1959   Mucopolysaccharides in human epidermis   Soc. Cosm. Chem. 10:
    154-158
Fly
1963   Tests of Aloe Vera for antibiotic activity   Economic Botony 17:46-
    49
Foster
1961   First Aid plant   The herb grower 14:16-23
Fox
Research paper
Fugita
1979   Properties of carboxupeptidase from Aloe   Biochemical
    Pharmacology 1997 28 1261-1262.
Fugita
1976   Bradykinase activity of Aloe extract Biochemical Parmacology 25:205
Fugita
1978   Specific reaction to Aloe extract   Experientia. 1978. 39. 523 - 524.
Fulton
1990   The stimulation of postermabrasion wound healing with stabilised A. V.
    gel-polyethylene oxide dressing. J. derm. Surg. Oncol. 1990 may 16(5). 460 -
    467.
Galban

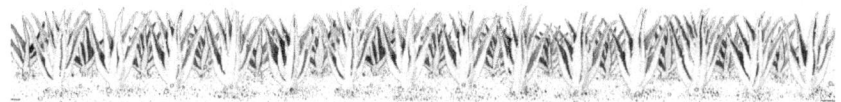

1952   Florida Herbs and plants   Herbarist 18:16-23
Garnick
1994   Changes in root sensitivity in toothpastes containing A. V. Archives of
     Oral Biology. 1994. 39. 132S.
Gates
1975   Aloe Vera - my favourite plant   Americal Horticulturis 54:37
Gerloff
1993   Study of the organoleptic properties of the exuded mucilage from the
     Aloe....   Technical info. on botanical and animal active ingredients for
     the cosmetic, perfumery and flavour industries. Aloe Vera. 1993. April-June.
Gjerstad
1969   An appraisal of the Aloe Vera Juice American Perfumer & Cosmetics
     84:43-46
Gjerstad
1968   Current status of Aloe as a cure all. Am. J. of Pharm. 1968. 140. 58 -
     64.
Gjerstad
1971   Chemical studies of Aloe Vera Juice   amino acid analysis, Adv.
     frontiers Plant Sci., 28: 311-315
Goff
1964   Measuring the effects of topical preparations upon the healing of skin
     wounds   Journal of the Society of Cosmetic Chemists 15:509-518
Goldberg
1944   The Aloe Vera plant   Achives of Dermatology & Syphilology 49:46
Gottlieb   Aloe Vera Heals
Gottshall
1949   The occurance of antibacterial substances active against M.
     tuberculosis in sed plants   Journal of clinical investigation 28:920-923
Gottshall
1950   Anti bacterial substances in seed plants active against tubercle bacilli.
     Am. Rev. Tuberc. 1950. 60. 475 - 480.
Gowda
1979   Structural studies of polysaccharides from Aloe Vera Carbohydrate
     Research 72:201-205
Grammer
1969   The effects of Aloe Vera Gel incorporated into dressing of tissue culture
     Masters thesis, Baylor University College of Dentistry. Dallas
Green
1996   Aloe Vera extracts in equine clinical practice. Veterinary Times. 1996
     Sept. 26(9) 16.
Grimminger
1993   Analytics of senna drugs with regard to the toxocological discussions of
     anthranoids   Pharmacology. 1993. Oct. 47 (Suppl. 1) 98 - 109.

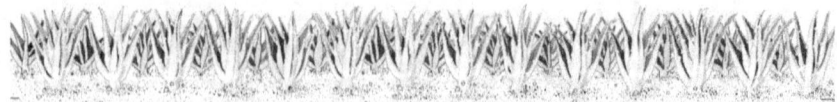

Grindley
1985   Medical use of Aloe Vera   General Practitioner London. Friday 14th
    June
Grindley
1985   Aloe Vera   The Garden Journal of the Royal Horticultural Society
    110:534-535
Gunther
1934   The Greek Herbal of Dioscorides   Oxford University Press
Hahn
1991   A natural polysaccharide having activity on the reticuloendothelial
    system from Aloe Vera exudate. Int. Congress of Phytotherapy. 1991. Oct.
    Seoul. Korea.
Haller
1990   A drug for all seasons, medical and pharmacological history of A. V.
    Bull. N.Y. Acad. Med. 1990. 66(6). 647 - 659. A14.
Harding
1979   Aloes of the World   Excelsa 9: 57-94
Harendal
1992   Whole leaf A. V.; almost a panacea.   Health Conscious. 1992.
    13(1). 14 - 17.
Harris
1991   Efficacy of acemannon in treatment of canine and feline spontaneous
    neoplasms.   Mol. Biother. 1991. 3. 207 - 213.
Harrison
1992   Aloe in dentistry   Health Concious. 1992. 13(1) 19 - 24.
Hart L. A.
1988   Two functionally and chemically distinct immuno-modulatory
    compounds in the gel of Aloe Vera   J Ethnopharmacol May-Jun 23 (1)
    61-71
Hart L. A. Van Den Barselaar M. T.
1990   Effects of low molecular constituents from Aloe Vera Gel on oxidative
    metabolism and cytotoxic and bacterial activities of human neutrophils
          Int J Immunopharmacol 12 (4) 427-434
Hart L. A. Van Den Berg A. J.
1989   An Anti-complementary polydassharide with immunological adjuvant
    activity from the leaf ... Gel of Aloe Vera
Heggers
Aloe and other topical anti bacterial agents in wound healing. Aloe today. Aloe
    Corp.. 1993. 8 - 11 - A4.
Heggers
1993   Beneficial effects of Aloe in wound healing.   Phytother. res. 1993. 7.
    S48 - 52.
Heggers

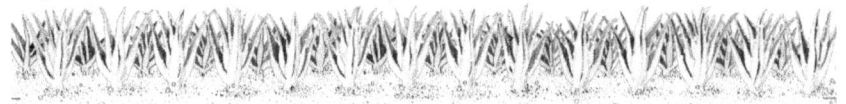

1966   Beneficial effects of Aloe in wound healing in an excisional wound
   model   J. of Alternative & Comp. Medicine. 1966. 2(20. 271 - 277.
Heggers
1991   The effect of oral administration of Aloe Vera gel extracts upon the
   induction of cysteamine induced gastric and duodenal ulcers in the male
   sprague dawley rat.   Int. Congress of Phytotherapy. 1991. Oct. Seol.
   Korea. 52.
Heggers
1997   Effect of the combination of A. V., nitroglycerine and L-name on wound
   healing in the rat excisional model.
Heidenmann
1996   Genotoxicity of Aloe Emodin in vitro and in vivo.   Mutat Res. 1996
   March. 367 (3). 123 - 133.
Heinerman
1982   Aloe Vera, the Divine Healer   J. of Alternative & Comp. Medicine.
   1967. 3(2). 149 - 153.
Henderson
Research paper
Henry
1979   An updated review of Aloe Vera   Cosmetics & Toiletries 94: 42-50
Henry
1991   Identification and standardisation of A. V. as a biological active
   ingredient for topical and internal products.   Int. Congress of
   Phytotherapy. 1991. Oct. Seoul. Korea. 57.
Hirata
1977   Biologically active constituents of leaves and roots of Aloe
          Zeitschrift 32:731-734
Hoffenburg
1979   The drug Aloes of commerce ....   Seifen..... 105:499-502
Holdsworth
1969   Chromones in Aloe Species   Plant Medicine 19:322-325
Horn
1941   Botanical science helps develop a new relief for human suffering
   Journal of the New York Botanical Garden 42:88-92
Ibo. S.
1991   Properties of pharmacological activity of carboxypeptidase in Aloe...
          Int. Congress of phytotherapy. 1991. Oct. seoul. Korea. 39.
Ibo. S.
1993   Biochemical properties of carboxypeptidase from Aloe.... Phytotherapy
   research 1993. 7.S26-29.
Imanishi
1991   An active substance of Aloe....   int. Congress of Phytotherapy.
   1991. Oct. Seoul Korea. 34.

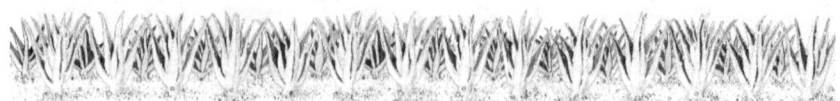

Imanishi K.
1993   Aloctin A. an active substance of Aloe arborescens Miller as immuno-
    modulator
Ishii
1990   Studies of Aloe III. Mech. of carthartic effect....   Chem. Pharm.
    Bull (Tokyo). 1990 Jan. 38(1). 197 - 200.
Ishii
1994   Studies of Aloe IV. Mech. of carthartic effect. Biol. Pharm. Bull. 1994.
    May. 17(5) 651 - 653.
Ishii
1994   Studies of Aloe Vera. Mech. of carthartic effect....   Biol. Pharm. Bull.
    1994. Apr. 17(4) 495 - 497.
Jeong
1994   Anticancer effects of Aloe on sarcoma 180 in ICR mouse and on human
    cancer cell lines   Yakhak Hoeji 1994. 38(3). 311 -321.
Joshi
1988   Hypoli[idaemic effect od Aloe barbadensis Aloe fraction I in cholesterol
    fed albino rats ....   Proc. Natl. Acad. Sci. India. SB (Biol. Sci.) 1988.
    56(4) 339-342.
Kahion
1991   Inhibition of aids virus replication by acemannan in vitro. Mol. Biother.
    1991. 3. 127 - 135.
Kahion
1991   In vitro evaluation of the synergistic antiviral effects of Acemannon.....
    Mol. Biother. 1991. 3. 214 - 223.
Karaca K.
1995   Nitric Oxide production by chicken macrophages activated by
    Acemannon   Int. J. Immuno pharmacol 17 (3) 183-188
Kaufman
1988   Aloe Vera gel hindered wound healing of experimantal second-degree
    burns; a quantitative controlled study.   j. Burn care rehabil. 1988 Mar-Apr.
    9(2), 156-159.
Kawai
1993   Tissue culture of Aloe B. M. var. nat. berger. Phytother. res. 1993. 7. S5
    - 10.
Khan
1983   Investigating the amino acid content of the exudate from the leaves of
    Aloe Barbadensis   Erde International 1:19-25
Klein
1988   Aloe Vera   J. of Am. Ac. Derm. 1988 18(4,1) 714 – 720
Knight. J. H.
1991   Anti-inflammatory and healing properties of Aloe....   Int. Congress of
    phytotherapy. 1991. Oct. Seoul. Korea. 31.

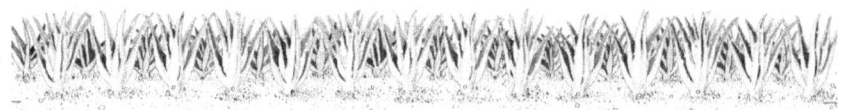

Koch
1993   Investigations of the laxative action of Aloin in the human colon. Planta
    Medica. 59 (Suppl. 7) 1993.
Koo
1994   A. V. anti-ulcer and anti-diabetic effects.   Phytother Res. 1994. 8(8).
    461 - 464.
Koshioka
1982   Studies on the evaluation of Aloe... International Journal of Crude Drug
    Research 20:53-59
Krumbiegel
1993   Rhein and Aloe-emodin kinetics from senna laxatives in man. Pharm.
    1993. Oct. 47(Suppl 1) 120 - 124.
Leung
1977   Aloe Vera in cosmetics   drugs & Cosmetic Industry 120:34-357
Leung
1978   Aloe Vera in cosmetics   Excelsa 8:65-68
Leung
1985   Aloe Vera update drug Cosmetic Ind. 1985. Sept. 137 - 42, 44 - 46.
Levene
1983   Medicine men hit town with cactus cure   Suday Times London 24th
    July
Levin
1988   Partial purification and some peroperties of an antibacterial compound
    from A. V.   Phytother. Res. 1988. 2(2) 67 - 69.
Lion Corp
1981   Cosmetics for Skin   Japanese Patent 80,104,205
Lorenzette.
1984   Bacteriostatic property of A. V.   Journal of Pharmaceutical Science.
    1984. 53. 1287.
Loveman
1937   Leaf of A.V. in the treatment of Roentgen Ray Ulcers. Archives of
    Dermatology and Syphilology 1937. 36. 838 - 843.
Lowenthal
1949   Species of Aloe in the treatment of Roentgen Dermatitis. The Journal of
    Investigative Dermatology 1949. 12. 295 - 298.
Lushbaugh
1953   Experimental acute radiodermatitis following beta radiation. V.
    histopthological study of the mode of action of therapy with Aloe VeraCancer
    6: 690-698
Madis Laboratories
1983   Aloe Vera   Cosmetics & Toiletries 98:99-104
Madis Laboratories

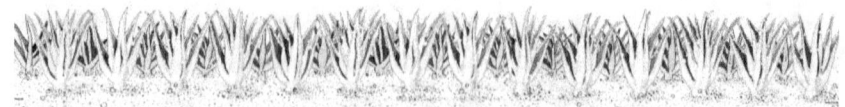

1984   Aloe Vera Gel, The Ageless beauty ingredient   9th edition Dr
    Madis Lab. Inc.
Mahmoud
1986   Microbiological studies on the phyliosphere of the desert plant A. V.
    1986. Egypt. J. Microbiol. 21(2) 229 - 238.
Malterud
1993   Antioxidant and radical scavenging effects of anthraquinones .... Pharm.
    1993. Oct. 47 (suppl 1.1) 77 - 85.
Mandal
1980   Structure of Glucomanan isolated from the leaves of Aloe Barbadensis
    Miller 87:249-256
Mandal
1980   Structure of the Dgalactan isolated from Aloe Barbadensis Miller
    86:247-257
Mandal
1983   Characterisation of polysaccharides of Aloe Barbadensis Miller
    22B:890-893
Mandeville
1939   Aloe Vera in the treatment of radiation ulcers of mucous membranes
    Radiology 32:598-599
Mapp
1970   The assessment of purgative principles in Aloes   Planta Medica
    18:361-365
Marshall
1990   Aloe Vera Gel, what is the evidence The Pharm. J. 1990. 360 - 362.
Marshall
1993   In vitro stimulation of NK activity by acemannon   J. Immunol.
    1993. 150. 1381.
Marshall
1993   Human cytokines induced by acemannon   J. Allergy Clin. Immunol.
    1993. 91. 295.
Martinet
1993   Preclinical and clinical evaluation of the cicatrizant effects of A. B.
    revista Farmaceutica (Argentina) 1993. 135. 101 - 106.
Maughan
1991   The Miracle of Aloe   The 20th World Congress of Natural
    Medicines, Madras India
Maykut
1995   Aloe Vera, The Health & Healing plant   Apophtegme ISBN 2-
    9508531
McAnalley
1988   U.S.Patent 4,735,935
McAnalley

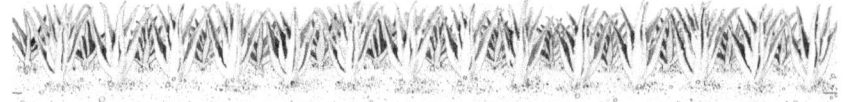

Uses of acemannon of other Aloe products in the treatment of diseases requiring intervention of the Immune System for cure. Carrington Laboratories Inc. USA. PCT. Int. Appl. 115. CODEN. PIXXD2.

McCarthy
1971 Aloe Research Aloe 9:20-23

McCarthy
1966 The seasonal variation of aloin in leaf juice from Aloe.... Planta Medica 14:62-65

McCarthy
1968 The metabolism of anthracene derivative & organic acids in selected Aloe species Plant Medicine 16: 348-356

McCauley
1990 Frostbite - methods to minimise tissue loss. Frostbite. 1990. 88(8). 72 - 77.

McDaniel
1987 Evolution of polymannoacetate in the treatment of AIDS. Clin. Res. 1987. 35. 483A.

McDaniel
1987 A clinical pilot study using Carrisyn TM in the treatment of aquired immunodeficiency syndrom (AIDS.) Ass. J. Clin. Pathol. 1987. 88 - 534.

McKeown
1987 Anthraquinones and anthracenic derivatives absorb .... 1987. June. 102. 64 - 65.

McKeown
1987 Aloe Vera Cosmetics and Toiletries 1987. 102. 64 - 65.

Meadows
1980 Aloes as a humectant in new skin preparations Cosmetics & Toiletries 95:51-56

Messa
1985 A study of the crude antidiabetic drugs used in Arabian folk medicine. Int. J. of crude drug research. 1985. 23(3). 137 - 145. A24.

Miller
1995 treatment of experimental frostbite with pentoxifylline and A. V. cream. Arch. Otolaringol heal neck surg. 1995 June. 121(6). 678 - 680.

Moroni
1982 Aloe in cosmetic formulations Cosmetic Technology Sept. 1982

Morrow
1980 Hypersensitivity to Aloe Archives of dermatology 116:1064-1065

Morsy
1993 Evaluating the healing characteristics of the exuded mucilage from A. B. j. of tech. info.on Botanical & Animal active ingredients for the cosmetic perfumery & flavour ind. 1993 June. 1. 1 - 80.

Mortaga

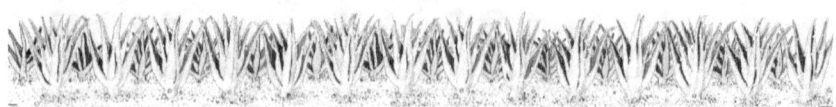

1976   Use of Aloe extracts in the treatment of experimental corneal ulcers
        Cs. Offal., 32(6) 424-427
Morton
1961   Folk uses and commercial exploitation of Aloe leaf pulp Economic
        Botony 15:311-319
Morton
1977   Aloe : in: Major Medicinal plants   Botony, Culture & Uses pp 46-50
Morton
1981   Atlas of medicinal plants of middle America   Springfield pp 78-80
Nakagomi
1985   A noval biological activity in Aloe components effects on mast cell
        degranulation and platelet aggregation.   Rep. Ferment. Res. Inst. (Yakabie)
        1985. 0(63). 23-30.
Nakasugi
1994   Antimutagen of Aloe plantsKinki Daigaku, Nogakubu, Kiyo. 1994. 27. 47
        - 54.
Nath
Commonly used Indian abortifacient plants with special reference to their
        teratologic effects in rats.   J. of Ethnopharmacol. 38(2) 147 - 159.
Natow
1986   Aloe Vera, fiction or fact.   Cutis. 1986. 37(2) 106 - 108.
Newton
1979   In defence of the name Aloe Vera   The Cactus and Succulent Journal
        of Great Britain 41:29-30
Norris
1973   The ancient wonder drug   Garden Journal new York Botanical Gardens
        23:172-173
Northway
Experimental use of Aloe Vera extract in clinical practice Veterinary
        Medicine/Small Animal Clinician 70,89
Nouri
1956   The effect of Some Selected Surface Active Agents on the Extraction of
        Cape Aloe.   J. Am. Pharm. Assoc. 1956. 45(6)
Obata M.
1993   Mechanism of anti-inflammatory and antithermal burn action of A. V.
        Phytother. res. 1993. 7. 530-533.
Odes
1991   A double blind trial of ... A. V. and psyllium laxative in adult patients with
        constipation.   Cosmetics and Toiletries. 1987 June. 102. 64 - 65
Oh, You-Jin.
1991   Effects of Aloe Vera... on cirrhosis patients.   Int. Congress of
        Phytotherapy. 1991. Oct. seoul. Korea. 42.

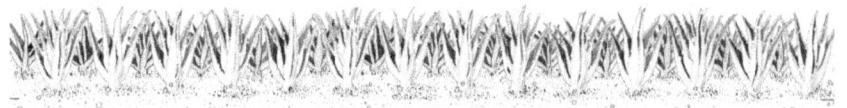

OSW, C. S.   1979   The effect of extracts of A. B. M. 11 leaves on the
   fertility of female rats.   Indian Drugs. 1979. 16(6). Mar. 127 - 135.
Ovodova
1975   Polysaccharides in Al;oe....   Khimija Prirodnykh Soedinenii 11:3-
   5
Parman
1986   Evaluation of Aloe Vera leaf exudate and gel for gastric and duodenal
   anti-ulcer activity.   Fitoterapia 57(5) 1986 380 - 383.
Parry
1992   Some pharm. actions of A. extracts ....   Cent. Afr. J. Med. 1992.
   Oct. 38(1C0 409 - 414.
Parry
1994   The uterine relaxant effect of Aloe.   Chapandi: Fitoterapia 1994. 65(3)
   253 - 259.
Patel
1986   Antibacterial activity of phenolic and nonphenolic fractions on some
   Indian medicinal plants. Indian drugs. 1986. 23(11) 595 - 597.
Paulsen
1978   Structural studies of polysaccharide from Aloe plicatilis Miller   60:345-
   351
Payne
1970   Tissue response to Aloe Vera Gel following Periodontal Surgery Thesis
   submitted .. Bayley University, for degree in Masters of Science
Pelley
1993   Current status of quality control of Aloe Barbadensis extracts SOFW
   Journal 255-268
Peng
1991   Decreased mortality of normal murine sarcoma in mice treated with the
   immunomodulator acemannon.   Mol. Biother. 1991. 3. 79 - 87.
Picker
Research paper
Pierce
1983   Comparison between the nutritional contents of the Aloe Vera Gel from
   conventional & hyproponically grown plants   Erde International 1:37-38
Pittman J. C.
1992   Immune enhancing effects of Aloe   Health Conscious 13 (1) 28-30
Plaskett L.
1997   The Exudate Compounds of Aloe Vera and their benefits biomedical
   Information Services Ltd
Plaskett L.
1997   Actiona of Aloe at Cellular Level and their relationship to nutrition
   biomedical Information Services Ltd
Plaskett L.

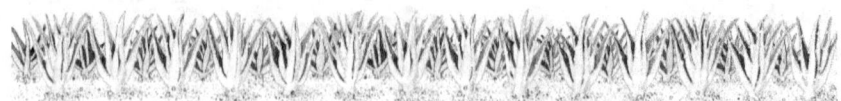

1997   The Carbohydrate Fraction of Aloe   biomedical Information Services Ltd
Plaskett L.   1
997   Aloe Vera and Sports Injuries   biomedical Information Services Ltd
Plaskett L.
1997   Aloe Vera Against Infections   biomedical Information Services Ltd

Plaskett L.
1997   Aloe Vera and Diabetes   biomedical Information Services Ltd
Plaskett L.
1997   Aloe Vera and Cancer   biomedical Information Services Ltd
Plaskett L.
1997   Aloe in Alternative Medicine Practice   biomedical Information
    Services Ltd
Plaskett L.
1997   Healing Properties of Aloe Vera   biomedical Information Services Ltd
Plaskett L.
1997   Aloe Vera and the Human Digestive system biomedical Information
    Services Ltd
Plaskett L.
1997   Aloe Vera and the Human Immune System   biomedical Information
    Services Ltd
Plemens
1994   Evaluation of acemannon in the treatment of recurrent aphthous
    stomatitis.   Wounds. 1994. 6(2) 40 - 45.
Proserpio
1976   Natural Sunscreens   Cosmetics & Toiletries 91:34-46
Radjabi
1983   Structural studies of glucomannon from Aloe Carbohydrate Research
    116:166-170
Rakatovao
1979   Mise en evidence et etude des proprietes immunostimulantes .....
    d'Aloe...   Archives de L'Instutute Pasteur de Madagasgar. 1979. 47. 9 -
    39.
Rauwald
1982   7 hydroxyaloin the leading substance from A. B. in European pharm.
        Arch. Pharm. 1982. 315(5). 477 - 478.
Reynolds
1950   The Aloes of South Africa The Trustees of the Aloes of South Africa
    Book Fund
Reynolds
1966   The Aloes of Tropical Africa & Madagascar   The Trustees of the Aloes
    of South Africa Book Fund
Reynolds

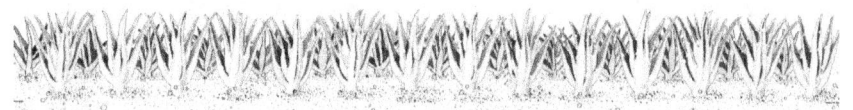

1985   The compounds in Aloe Leaf exudates   The Trustees of the Aloes
    of South Africa Book Fund
Reynolds
1985   Observations on the phytochemistry of the Aloe leaf exudate
    compounds.   Botanical J. Linnean Society. 1985. 90. 179 - 199.
Ritter
1993   Aloe Vera A Mission Discovered   Triputic. ISBN 0 9638609 0 9
Roberts
1995   Acemannon containing wound dressing gel reduces radiation-induced
    skin reactions in C3H mice.   Int. J. Radiation Oncol. Biol. Phys.
1995. 32(4) 1047 - 1052.
Roboz
1948   A mucilage from Aloe Vera Journal of the Americal Journal Society
    70:3248-3249
Robson
1979   Myth, magic, witchcraft or fact? Aloe Vera revisited.   American burn
    association abstracts 31:65-66
Rodriguez-Bigas.
1988   Comparative evaluation of A. V. in the management of burn wounds in
    guinea pigs.   Plast. Reconstr, surg. (U.S.) 1988. 81(3). 386 - 389.
Roman Ramos.
1991   Experimental study of the hypoglycaemic effect of some antidiabetic
    plants.   Arch. Invest. Med. Mex. 1991 Jan-Mar. 22(1) 87 - 93.
Rovatti
1959   Experimental thermal burns   Industrial Medicine & Surgery
    28:364-368
Rowe
1940   Effect of fresh Aloe Vera jelly in the treatment of third degree Roentgen
    reaction in white rats   Journal of the American Pharmaceutical Association
    29:348-350
Rowe
1941   Phytochemical study of Aloe Vera Leaf   Journal of the American
    Pharmaceutical Association 30:262-266
Rowe
1941   Further observations on the use of Aloe Vera leaf in the treatment of
    third degree Xray reactions   Journal of the American Pharmaceutical
    Association 30:266-269
Rowson
1967   The chemical assay of Aloes   Analyst 92:593-596
Rubel
1983   Possible mechanisms of the healing actions of Aloe Gel
        Cosmetics & Toiletries 98:109-114
Saga

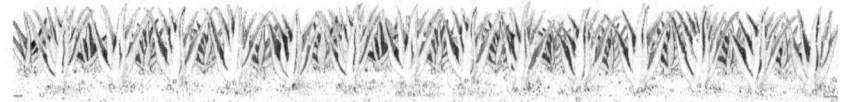

1983   The efficacy of the Aloe plants   Cosmet. Toiletries. 1983. 98105 -
    108.
Saito
1982   Pharmacological studies on a plant lectin Aloctin   Japanese Journal
    of Pharmacology 32:139-142
Schmidt
1991   A. V. dermal wound gel is associated with a delay in wound healing.
    Obstet. Gynaecol (U.S.) 1991 July 78(1). 115 - 117.
Segal
1968   A re-investigation of the polysaccharide material from Aloe Vera
    mucliage   Lloydia 31:423
Sendelbach
1989   Review of the toxicity and Carcinogenicity of Anthraquinine derivatives
    Toxicology 1989. 57. 277 - 240.
Shahmaz
1993   Aloe, a biologically active & potential medicinal plant. Hamdard
    Medicus. 1993. 36(1) 108 - 115.
Sharma
1997   Phytochemical synergism: beyond the active ingredient model.
    Alternative Therapies in Clinical practice. 1997. 4(3). 91 - 96.
Sheets M. A.
1991   Studies on the effect of Acemannon on retrovirus infections: clinical
    stabilization of feline virus infected cats   Mol. Biother. 3 41-45
Shelton
1991   A. V. its chemical & therapeutical properties. Int. journal of dermatology.
    1991. 30. 679 - 683.
Ship
1977   Is topical Aloe Vera plant mucus helpful in burn treatment?   Journal
    of the American Medical Association 238:1770
Siegers
1993   Sennosides and Aloin do not promote dimethylhydrazine-induced
    tumours in mice.   pharm. 1993. Oct. 47. (Suppl. 7) 205 - 208.
Siegers
1993   Anthranoid laxative abuse - a risk for colorectal cancer? Gut. 1993.
    Aug. 34(8) 1099 - 1101.
Sims
1971   Effectiveness of undiluted Aloe99 Gel against Trichomonas Vaginalis...
    Aloe Vera od America Archives. Stabilised A.V. 1971. 1. 241 - 242..
Sims
Report on the effect of Aloe Vera on growth of certain micro-organisms. Baylon
    College of Dentistry, Dallas Microb Assay Services. 1969. 1. 230 - 233.
Sims

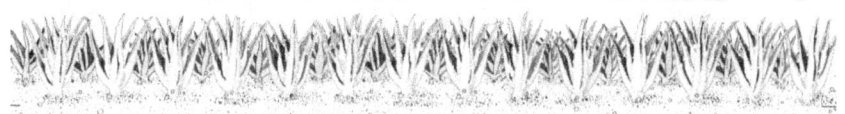

1971   Effect of A. V. on Herpes Simplex....Aloe Vera od America Archives.
    Stabilised A.V. 1971. 1. 239 - 240.
Sims
1971   The effects of A. V. on Mycotic Organisms (Fungi).   Aloe Vera od
    America Archives. Stabilised A.V. 1971. 1. 237 - 238.
Skousen
1982   Aloe Vera Handbook   Aloe Vera Research Institute. 5103 Sequoia.
    Cyprus. CA 90630
Skousen
1977   Aloe Vera Quotations from Medical Journals Aloe Vera Research
    Institute. 5103 Sequoia. Cyprus. CA 90630
Soeda
    1966 Studies on anti-bacterial and anti-fungal activity of Cape Aloe   Nippon
    Saikingaku Zasshi 1966. 21. 609 - 619.
Spoerke
1980   Aloe Vera - fact or quackery   Vet. & Human Toxicology. 1980.
    22. 418 - 429.
Suga
1983   The efficacy of the Aloe plant chemical constituents & biologicl activities
    Cosmetics & Toiletries 98:105-108
Sumano Lopez
    1989 Comparative evaluation of a mixture of propolis and A. V. with
        commercial wound healing products. Veterimarcia Mexico 1989 20(4).
        408 - 414.
Swain
1992   Effects of topical medications on the healing of open pad wounds in
    dogs. J. of the Am.Animal Hosp. Assoc. 1992. 28(6). 499 - 502.
Sydiskis
1989   Inactivation of Herpes simplex virus by Anthraquinones isolated from
    plants   J Dental Res. 1989. June. 68. 935.
Sydiskis
1991   Inactivation of enveloped viruses by anthraquinones extracted from
    plants.   Antimicrob-Agents-Chemother. 1991. Dec. 35(12) 2463 - 2466.
Syed
1997   Management of genital herpes in men with 5% A. V. extract in a
    hydrophilic cream... aplacebo controlled double blind study. Journal of
    Dermatological Treatment. 1997. 8. 99 - 102.
Syed
1996   Management of psoriasis with A. V. cream... tropical med. & Int. Health.
    1996. 1(4) 505 - 509.
Taylor
1980   Aloe Vera "Wand of Heaven"   Bestways
Taylor

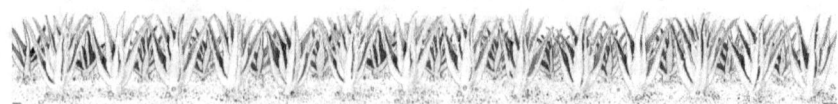

1981   A runners guide to discovering the secrets of Aloe Vera plant   Runners
World Dec. 1981
Tchou
1943   Aloe Vera   Archives of Derm. & Syph. 1943. 47. 249.
Teradaira
1993   Antigastric ulcer effects in rats of Aloe ....   Phytother. Res. 1993. 7.
534 - 536.
Terry Corporation
Texas Aloe Florida Style   Terry Corp. Melbourne. Florida
Thomlinson
1980   Kitchen remedy for necrotic malignant breast ulcers.   Lancet. 1980. 2:
707.
Tizard
1993   Accelerated wound healing induced by macrophage stimulants in rats: a
genetically controlled phenomenon.   Wound Repair and Regeneration.
1993. 1. 130.
Tizard
1991   Immuno-regulatory effects of a cytokine release enhancer
(acemannon). Int. Cong. of Phytotherapy. 1991. Oct. seoul. Korea. 68.
Tolbert
1997   Aloe Vera, past present and future   Seigen, Oele, Fette, Wachse
(Germany) 1997 Jan. 120. 14 - 18.
Trease
1978   Pharmacognosy   Balliere Tindall London
Tsuda
1993   Inhibitory effect of Aloe ..... on induction of preneoplastic focal lesions in
the rat liver.   International Congress of Phytotherapy. 1991. Oct. Seoul.
Korea 53.
Tyler
Aloe, the honest Herbal
Udupa S. L.
1994   Anti-inflammatory and wound healing properties of A. V. Fitoterapia
1994. 65(2) 141-145.
Vagi
1982   Cardiac stimulant action of constituents of Aloe...   J. of
Pharmaceutical Sciences. 1982a. 71. 739 - 741.
Visuthikosol
1993   Effect of A. V. Gel on healing of burn wound. J. Med. Assoc. Thai. 1995
78(8) 403 - 409. A21
Visuthikosol
1995   Effect of A. V. Gel on healing of burn wound a clinical and histologic
study.   J. Med. Assoc. Thai. 1993 Aug. 78(8). 703 - 709.
Waller

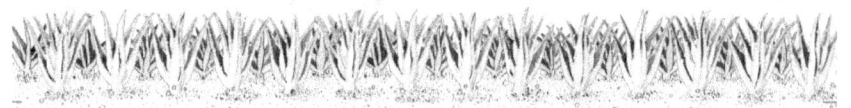

86

Quality control, biological activity of Aloe B. extracts. CTMW 64-80
Waller
1978   A chemical investigation of Aloe Barbadensis Miller   Proceedings of
    the Oklahoma Academy of Science 58:69-76
Waller
Aloe Vera   A publication of Aloe Vera Products Inc. New Mexico
Wang
1991   Monitoring physical and chemical properties of freshly harvested field
    grown A. V. leaves.   Phytother. Res. 1993 7 Spec. Issue. proceedings of
    the Int. Congress of Phytotherapy. 1991. S1 - 4.
Watcher
    1989 The role of topical agents in the healing of full thickness wounds. j.
        Derm. Surg. Oncol. 1989 Nov. 15(11). 1188 - 1195.
Westendorf
1990   Genotocicity of natural occuring Hydroxyanthraquinones. Evaluation of
    Mutagenicity and cell transforming activity Mutat. Res. 1990 Jan. 240(1) 1 - 12
Williams
1996   Phase III double blind evaluation of A. V. Gel as a prophylactic agent for
    radiation induced skin toxicity.   Int. J.Radiation. Oncol-Biol-Phys. 1996 sept
    36(2) 345 - 349.
Wimbus
1981   Effects of Aloe extracts on human tumour cells in-vitro Econ. Bot. 1981.
    35(1) 89 - 95
Winters
1981   Effects of Aloe extracts on human normal & tumour cells in vitro
    Economic Botony 35:89-95
Winters W. D.
1993   Immunoreactive Lectins in Leaf Gel from Aloe Barbadensis Miller
        Phytotherapy Research 7 523-525
Wolfe
1990   Hydroxyanthraquinones as tumour promoters: enhancement of
    malignant transformation of C3H mouse fibroblasts and growth stimulation
        Cancer Res. (USA). 1990 Oct. 50(20). 6540 - 6544.
Womble D.
1988   Enhancement of Allo-Responsiveness of Human Lymphocytes by
    Acemannan   Panta Med 55 (6) 509 - 12
Womble D.
1992   The impact of acemannon on the generation and function of cytotoxic T-
    lymphocytes.   Immunopharmacol Imm. 1992. 14. 63 - 77.
Wood
1983   The Aloes of the Yemen Arab Republic   Kew Bulletin 38:13-31
Wright

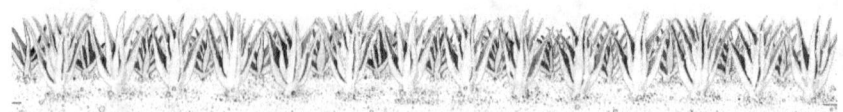

1936   A. V. in the treatment of Roentgen Ulcers and Telangientasis.   Journal of the Am. Med. Assoc. 1936. 106. 1363 - 1364.

Yagi
1977   Aloe mannan, polysaccharide from Aloe   31:17-20

Yagi
1982   Antibradykinin active material in Aloe saponaria   Journal of Pharmaceutical Sciences 71:1172-1174

Yagi
1984   Structural determination of polysaccharides in Aloe... Journal of Pharmaceutical Sciences 73: 62-65

Yagi
1985   Effect of Aloe Extract on Peripheral Phogocytosis in Adult Bronchial Asthma   Planta Med. pp273-275

Yagi
1987   Effect of Amino Acids in Aloe Extract on Phogocytosis by peripheral neutrophils in Adult Bronchial Asthma   Jpn J. Allergol 36 (12) 1094-1101

Yamaguchi
1993   Components of the gel of Aloe Vera.   Biosci. Biotechnol. Biochem. 1993 Aug. 57.(8) 1350 - 1352.

Yamamoto
1993   Inhibitory effects of Aloe extracts on antigen ....   Japanese Journal of Toxicology and environmental Health. 1993. 39(5) 395-400

Yamoto
1993   Formulating beverage products from stabilised Aloe.   j. of Tech. Inf. on botanical & animal active ing. for the cosmetic and perfumery and flavouring industry. 1993. Apr. - June. 1(1) 1 - 80.

Yaron
1991   Characteristics of Aloe Gel...   Phytother. of Phytotherapy. 1991. S11 -13.

Yongchaiyudia
1996   Antidiabetic activity of A. V. juice I. Clinical trial in new cases of diabetes mellitus.   Phytomedicine. 1996. 3(3) 241 - 243.

Yongchaiyudia
1996   Antidiabetic activity of A. V. juice II. Clinical trial in new cases of diabetes mellitus.   Phytomedicine. 1996. 3(3) 245 - 248.

Zawahry El
1973   Use of Aloe in treating leg ulcers and dermatoses International Journal of Dermatology 12:68-73

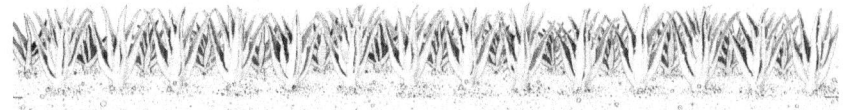